Fabiano José da Silva Boulhosa
Aurimery Gomes Chermont
Rafaela Cordeiro de Macêdo

Avoidability of neonatal death in low birth weight premature infants in the ICU

Fabiano José da Silva Boulhosa
Aurimery Gomes Chermont
Rafaela Cordeiro de Macêdo

Avoidability of neonatal death in low birth weight premature infants in the ICU

ScienciaScripts

Imprint

Cover image: www.ingimage.com

This book is a translation from the original published under ISBN 978-613-9-64217-5.

Publisher:
Sciencia Scripts
is a trademark of
Dodo Books Indian Ocean Ltd. and OmniScriptum S.R.L publishing group

120 High Road, East Finchley, London, N2 9ED, United Kingdom
Str. Armeneasca 28/1, office 1, Chisinau MD-2012, Republic of Moldova, Europe
Printed at: see last page
ISBN: 978-620-7-76266-8

To my mum, who has always been by my side at all times.

ACKNOWLEDGEMENTS

To God for giving me the gift of life, health and discernment to fulfil all my academic goals.

To my parents for always encouraging me to study under any circumstances.

To Rafaela, who has always been by my side, in moments of euphoria and regret, never lacking in sweet words aimed at the best direction for my life.

To Dr Aurimery Gomes Chermont, an example of humility, wisdom and love. Thank you for all your guidance in this work, always with patience, wit and astuteness.

To my family for always being my role models.

My letter of intent and entry into the programme would not have been the same without your help (Professor Leny Silene Castro and my on-call friend Kelly Costa).

To Patrícia Gazel, Paola Estesves and Samyra Said for their great contribution to the theoretical framework.

To the students Cinthia, Daniella, Dhyellen and Luã. Without you, data collection would have been miserable.

To the experts in biostatistics, everything became clearer after their analyses and comments (Professor Helder Pinheiro and Professor Renato Teixeira).

To my work colleagues for helping me find the time to carry out the research.

Sidney Monteiro and Fernanda Gomes for making the product.

To my classmates in the master's programme, the course would have been very monotonous without all of you.

To the professors of the programme, without the modules we would still be in the same place.

"As soon as love entered the middle, the middle became love, the fire melted, the ice ignited, and the breeze that was a typhoon, after the sea spilled, after the house fell, the wind of peace blew!"
Marcelo Camelo

SUMMARY

BOULHOSA, F.J.S. **Preventability of neonatal death in very low birth weight premature infants admitted to the Intensive Care Units of a teaching hospital in the Northern Region.** 2016. Dissertation (Professional master's degree in management and health services in the Amazon) - Santa Casa de Misericórdia do Pará Foundation FSCMPA, 2016.

INTRODUCTION: Analysing neonatal intensive care units, low birth weight is an important cause of morbidity and mortality. Researchers point out that knowledge of the population treated in hospital services can subsidise health care actions, meeting their needs and planning efficient care. **OBJECTIVE To** analyse the clinical, epidemiological and socio-demographic profile of premature newborns (NBs) weighing less than or equal to 1,500g admitted to Intensive Care Units (ICUs) in 2014. **METHODOLOGY An** analytical, comparative and retrospective study of the profile of NBs under/equal to 1,500g admitted to the ICUs of a school hospital in the northern region of Portugal. Discharge/death outcome factors were subjected to multivariate analysis. **RESULTS** The study population consisted of 248 records of NBs weighing less than or equal to 1,500g, of which 176 (71%) met the inclusion criteria and 72 (29%) were excluded. The average maternal age was 25.06 years. As for origin, more than half of the mothers 105 (59.65%) came from the interior of the state. With regard to prenatal care, the majority had incomplete prenatal visits. The predominant gender was male (97/ 55.11%). The average gestational age was 29.85 weeks and the average weight was 955g. The use of vasoactive drugs was applied in 157 (90%). Sedation/analgesia was used in 119 (67.61%) patients. Mechanical ventilation via tracheal tube was the most prevalent form of ventilatory support, with 162 (92.04%). The average length of ICU stay was 13.15 days. ICU stays of up to seven days had the highest frequency at 98 (55.68%). Of the neonates hospitalised, 171 (97.15%) had some kind of complication. It was also observed that the frequency of infection was 106 (60.22%) and of these the most frequent site of infection was the bloodstream 51 (48.11%). Discharge due to death was the most common, with 142 (80.68%), and pulmonary haemorrhage dominated the death report with 58 (40.85%). As for the variables correlated with the discharge/death outcome, statistical significance was found in relation to low weight, length of stay and use of surfactant in the delivery room, with greater chances of NBs dying. **CONCLUSION:** The lower the NBs' weight, the greater the chances of death due to various complications. In other words, the lower the weight, the more medication was used. However, despite the data, there was no increase in the length of stay in the units and/or a reduction in the mortality rate. In this context, we can see the fragility of health services in relation to the care of low birth weight neonates in ICUs and the need to apply new routines and continuing education, so that neonates can survive longer and with better results. **PRODUCT: This** will consist of a multi-professional bedside visit protocol aimed at improving communication between all the professionals involved with premature babies.
Keywords: Low birth weight, Neonatology, Intensive care unit.

SUMMARY

CHAPTER 1

INTRODUCTION

In the 1800s, the majority of the population was treated by the family doctor, and hospitals were of little relevance to society, so until the end of the 19th century, the concept was that these institutions offered no care beyond what was done at home (UNGERER; MIRANDA, 1999). At that time, hospitals were seen as shelters exclusively for the indigent, where the art of caring was practised without specific techniques or training for care (BENEVIDES; PASSOS, 2004).

Also in the 19th century, births took place in homes, with the midwife surrounded by relatives, and newborns were kept close to their mothers immediately after birth. According to Ungerer and Miranda (1999) the first nursery was created in 1893 in Paris.

The history of the emergence of Neonatology is told by AVERY (1984) in his book "Neonatology, Physiology and Treatment of the Newborn". According to this author, Neonatology as a speciality emerged in France. Obstetrician Dr Pierre Budin decided to extend his concerns beyond the delivery room and created the Childcare Outpatient Clinic at the Charité Hospital in Paris in 1882. Later, he headed a Special Department for the Debilitated established at the Maternity Hospital by Madame Hery, the former head midwife. In 1914, the first centre for premature newborns was created by a paediatrician, Dr Julius Hess, at the Michel Reese Hospital in Chicago. After that, several other centres were set up, following the principles of obstetrician Dr Budin and paediatrician Dr Hess, for the segregation of premature newborns with the aim of providing them with trained nurses, their own devices, including incubators, and strict procedures for preventing infections (ALMEIDA, 2011).

It was in Denmark, after a polio crisis in 1950, that the possibility of allocating more seriously ill patients to specific and more appropriate places was first considered, and the need was realised for professionals working in these sectors to have more specific knowledge, such as intensive care physicians. Currently, intensive care units (ICUs) are places that correspond to 5-10% of the beds in a hospital, designed to meet the demands of critically ill patients who require continuous monitoring and are assisted by a multidisciplinary team (ULTRA, 2009).

The intensive care unit stands out and differs from other hospital environments because it seeks to maintain life and rehabilitate the clinical condition of patients through intensive care. For this to happen, the team must be integrated and the professionals who work in it must be properly qualified (NASCIMENTO; JARDIM, 2013).

The neonatal period, between birth and the first 28 days of life, is a time of great fragility in a child's life, concentrating environmental, biological, cultural and socio-economic risks and therefore requiring special, comprehensive and qualified care. In addition, their health conditions are directly related to the conditions of their mothers during prenatal care, labour and the puerperium (UNICEF, 2009; BASSO *et al,* 2012; BRASIL, 2012; SBP, 2012).

According to Carmo *et al* (2004), admission to the Neonatal Intensive Care Unit consists of receiving a newborn baby who has difficulties adapting to extra-uterine life or pathologies that interfere with their survival, offering them special care and technologies through a multi-professional team with technical skills and clinical experience, organisation, procedures and protocols aimed at their stability.

Analysing the demand for Neonatal Intensive Care Units, low birth weight is one of the most important causes of morbidity and mortality, considering the increasing rates of poorly managed pregnancies due to poor socioeconomic conditions, maternal age, low maternal weight at the beginning of pregnancy, smoking, emotional instability at the time of pregnancy and poor prenatal care. According to the World Health Organisation (WHO, 2014), underweight is one of the most significant indicators of a child's quality of life.

According to data from the SUS Information Technology Department (DATASUS) in 2013, there were 41,638 hospitalisations in Intensive Care Units in the state of Pará, of which 5,409 were reported in neonatal units.

Granzotto *et al* (2012) point out that knowledge of the population cared for in hospital services, especially in NICUs, made available through appropriate epidemiological studies, can support health care actions, organising them, better meeting their needs and planning more efficient care.

However, according to Gomes (2004), there is still a great distance between what is advocated by public health policies and real life, resulting in inadequate maternal and child care, from the most basic levels of care to those of greater structural complexity, such as the NICU.

In collaboration with this, Rocha *et al* (2011) and the Ministry of Health (2012) point out that knowledge and analysis of birth conditions and neonatal deaths, as well as biological information on pregnancy and childbirth, the frequency of caesarean sections, prematurity, maternal age and schooling, low birth weight and birth asphyxia also make it possible to construct epidemiological data showing the real quality of maternal and child care, guiding the planning of actions in health services.

According to Costa *et al* (2014), vital events are processes inherent to life. However, birth, growth, illness and death, however natural they may seem, do not occur without at least one cause. From this perspective, birth weight can be understood as an indicator of gestational conditions, and more specifically of intrauterine growth, and can also be an important risk marker for infant morbidity and mortality.

In this context, this study aims to analyse the profile of newborns weighing less than or equal to 1,500g in a neonatal intensive care unit, relating their morbidity and mortality, length of stay and weight variations in a reference hospital located in the metropolitan region of Belém-Pará.

CHAPTER 2

BACKGROUND

With improvements and technological innovations in healthcare, Intensive Care Units have emerged with the aim of promoting patient safety through continuous vigilance on the part of the professionals who work there (FAVARIN; COMPONOGARA, 2012).

In Brazil there are 25,367 beds divided into 2,342 ICUs in 403 cities, registered with DATASUS. However, these figures are far from ideal, as it is estimated that three ICU beds are needed for every 10,000 inhabitants and in this country the coverage is less than half of what is desired, with only 1.3 beds for every 10,000 inhabitants (VIEIRA, 2011).

Among the neonatal population, premature and low birth weight newborns represent the groups most vulnerable to death, as well as generating longer hospital stays. Low birth weight and the factors associated with this condition are fundamental in planning public health and nutrition programmes and policies (VIANA, 2013).

The frequency of preterm births and low birth weight newborns is high all over the world. This neonatal population is the group most vulnerable to death, with very low birth weight NBs, i.e. those with a birth weight of less than 1,500 g, contributing the most to the rise in mortality, responsible for approximately 25 to 30 per cent of infant mortality and 50 to 70 per cent of neonatal mortality. (FIGUEIRÓ FILHO, 2014)

For Favarin and Componogara (2012), it is necessary to know the profile of these users admitted to Intensive Care Units in order to have data that allows for better planning of the patient's overall care. This knowledge is necessary because it enables strategies to be drawn up to better assist the individuals admitted, assessing their prognosis, the effects of the therapy implemented, as well as the risk factors that make them vulnerable.

According to data from DATASUS, Pará has been the leader in perinatal mortality, with 15/1000, and there is only one public maternity hospital in the capital that attends high-risk births, most of which come from the interior. So the Santa Casa de Misericórdia do Pará Foundation (FSCMPA) has 120 beds in shared accommodation, 60 intermediate care units and 60 Neonatal Intensive Care Unit. According to the institution's own data, an average of 700 children are born every year and of these, according to the statistics department, 18 per cent are underweight or very underweight. Although the intensive care unit has very few beds in the hospital, the financial resources allocated to it are extremely high. A day in a single NICU bed at FSCMPA costs an average of R$2,500.00 (two thousand five hundred reais), according to data from the finance department.

Thus, knowledge of the morbidity and mortality associated with very low birth weight in the institution is of fundamental importance for implementing measures that result in favourable indicators and improved survival for this population.

Thus, analysing the importance of Intensive Care Units for health care, it is necessary to characterise the population admitted and the effects of the treatments used there. In this context, the possibility of improving the care provided and minimising the risks exposed to the patient should be mandatory for any service working with critically ill newborns.

CHAPTER 3

OBJECTIVES

1.1- GENERAL OBJECTIVE

- To analyse the clinical, epidemiological and socio-demographic profile of premature newborns weighing less than or equal to 1,500 g admitted to Intensive Care Units (ICUs) from January to December 2014.

1.2- SPECIFIC OBJECTIVES

- To analyse the length of stay of neonates in ICUs.
- Show the different weight ranges of less than or equal to 1,500g, with length of stay and morbidity and mortality.
- To identify whether there is a relationship between length of stay and comorbidities with the use of medication.
- Correlate length of stay and/or ventilatory support.
- To verify the mortality rate and its probable relationship with the antimicrobials used during the ICU stay.
- Proposing the unification of neonatal care in the different ICUs through protocols discussed during shifts.

CHAPTER 4

THEORETICAL FRAMEWORK

4.1 Epidemiology in Health Services Management

According to Bonita *et al* (2010) epidemiology can be conceptualised as the study of the distribution and determinants or causes of health-related states or events in a given human population in a given region or over a period of time, and its application to the prevention and control of health problems.

For almost half a century, epidemiology has been used to describe disease in the community, identify risk groups and evaluate health services and programmes. However, the establishment of epidemiology as a scientific discipline and the epistemological reflection on it followed their own paths for some time, without any kind of more substantial link to the social organisation of health services, given the relative autonomy of the scientific fields (PAIM, 2003).

According to Alves, 2008, epidemiology, as technological knowledge, can be investigated in its application as a tool for policy formulation, planning and health evaluation. Health services, on the other hand, much more orientated towards the logic of the market than health needs, did not seem to see epidemiology as a necessary tool for their development. In this sense, we saw the possibility of making rational use of the concepts and possibilities arising from epidemiology in order to be able to plan targeted actions based on real scenarios - which would certainly contribute to better resolution in the health field. (ALVES, 2008)

In general, epidemiological research for health services has the following objectives: to study the occurrence, distribution and progression of health problems in a given human population, as well as their determinants and trends, in order to provide a basis for planning, evaluating and managing health promotion and disease prevention; epidemiological surveillance of diseases and other health problems; providing data that contributes to understanding the aetiology of health and disease, in order to promote causal and explanatory research into priority health problems; evaluating the impact on health of services, programmes, technologies and other actions aimed at this end; and through these, promoting the use of epidemiological concepts for the management of health services (DEVER;

CHAMPAGNER, 1988; BONITA *et al,* 2010; PAIM, 2003).

According to Paim (2003), over the last few decades various international organisations have advocated the creation of health services based on the concepts of epidemiology and management in the formulation of public health policies, defining priorities, objectives, strategies and interventions in professional practice, in research priorities and the allocation of resources and in the preparation of diagnoses and analyses of the health situation in order to produce changes in the epidemiological profile and incorporate surveillance actions in all health care units, including hospitals.

In this way, epidemiology can and should be used as an instrument of transformation. As the concepts of epidemiology are incorporated into the management of health services, it can be seen that transformations are gradually taking place, transforming a simple routine into an instrument of feedback to the community, through the Health Councils, health professionals and workers in general. Having said this, we realise that epidemiology has the capacity to transcend administrations and that, as a science, it has permanent status, despite changes in government. In order to transform, it is necessary to identify, interpret and use data effectively in decision-making (ROUQUAYROL, SILVA, 1998).

In Brazil, epidemiology has been recognised as a strategic mechanism in the construction and consolidation of the Unified Health System (SUS), through the documents that constitute its legal foundation, with the use of epidemiology described in the Organic Health Law (8.080/90) as one of its principles and guidelines "in the establishment of priorities, allocation of resources and programmatic orientation".

It can also be seen from the health sector that, despite being included in official documents, the use of epidemiology still falls short of its potential, due to factors such as the quantitative and qualitative shortage of trained human resources and the failure to take epidemiological information into account when defining health policies and actions - the latter, however, has recently shown a tendency to change (FERREIRA, BRANCO, 2005).

According to Rocha *et al* (2011), the epidemiological information available on the conditions of pregnancy and newborns, prenatal care and childbirth, causes of death and their avoidability is fundamental for planning strategies aimed at improving them, as well as contributing to the organisation of local intervention programmes and the quality of health care.

In Brazil, the development and implementation of public policies on maternal and child health began in the 1970s, with the aim of reducing morbidity and mortality. Initiatives were formulated and implemented for food supplementation, vaccination coverage, care for pregnant women, childbirth and family planning, and child and adolescent health care. Some of the programmes created continued, were reformulated and expanded, and some are still in force today (FERRARI *et al,* 2014).

Studies show that from the 1980s onwards, the relationship between maternal and child policies and programmes instituted to reduce mortality rates, despite their limitations, reflected an improvement in neonatal mortality indicators. However, little progress has been made in implementing public policies that favour better maternal health care (FERRARI *et al,* 2014)

In line with global trends, there has been a reduction in infant mortality in Brazil, but this trend has not been as marked in neonatal mortality, suggesting shortcomings in the quality of obstetric and neonatal care. The quality of care offered to mothers and newborns during the prenatal, labour and neonatal periods is reflected in the neonatal element of infant mortality (SILVA *et al,* 2014).

Adequate care during pre-pregnancy, pregnancy, childbirth and the newborn are considered essential interventions for promoting neonatal health. However, profound national and regional inequalities, limited access to the necessary care, inequality in the distribution of neonatal intensive care beds and the fragility of the services provided contribute as factors associated with the risk of neonatal death (SILVA *etal,* 2014).

Granzotto *et al* (2012) emphasise that knowledge of the population cared for in neonatal health services and the factors involved make it possible to plan the most appropriate care for this public, especially in cases requiring hospitalisation in Neonatal Intensive Care Units.

Finally, the availability of adequate epidemiological information allows for a change in the profile of actions, intervening directly in care processes and meeting the current needs of health services, particularly Neonatal Intensive Care Units, making it effective for organising and evaluating the various levels that make it up (BRASIL, 2009).

4.2 Maternal and Neonatal Care

According to the World Health Organisation, the neonatal period is from the moment a child is born until it is 28 days old (BRASIL, 2011, A).

This period can be understood as a time of great vulnerability in a child's life, when biological, environmental, socio-economic and cultural risks are concentrated and there is therefore a need for special, comprehensive and qualified care, social protection, health and rights (BRASIL, 2012, A).

In addition, the health conditions of the mother and her child are intrinsically linked. Therefore, the implementation of prenatal interventions, specialised care at the time of childbirth, access to emergency obstetric care and care for the newborn are actions that guarantee a better health condition for this binomial and the minimisation of its problems (UNICEF, 2009; BASSO *et al,* 2012; BRASIL, 2012 A, C; SBP, 2012).

As far as neonatal care is concerned, it was only in the 19th and early 20th centuries that institutionalised care for this population began to emerge, mainly in European countries and the United States, with the introduction of the first nurseries for premature babies, incorporating scientific and technological practices and knowledge to replace the work of midwives (SCOCHI; COSTA; YAMANAKA, 1996; ROSA; GAÍVA, 2009).

These advances in care, followed by several countries, led to an increase in births in hospital beds, thus triggering the creation of spaces to care for neonates and the increasingly advanced use of technology and human resources to assist them, with nurseries gradually being replaced by Joint Accommodation Units, Neonatal Intermediate Care Units (NICUs) and Neonatal Intensive Care Units (NICUs), enabling the survival of children previously considered unviable due to prematurity and low birth weight, and gradually reducing neonatal mortality (KAMADA; ROCHA; BARBEIRA, 2003; MOREIRA; LOPES, 2004; ASSIS, 2008; CLOHERTY *et al,* 2009; TRONCO *et al,* 2010).

Currently, hospital care for newborns involves a physical structure based on various spaces and levels of care, which start in the Obstetric Centre and are complemented by the Joint Accommodation and the Neonatal Intensive Care Unit (NICU), contributing to adequate care for the child (ROSA; GAÍVA, 2009).

With regard to antenatal care, the Ministry of Health (2012) presupposes that antenatal care should be carried out as a dynamic assessment of maternal and foetal risk situations and the readiness to act in order to prevent an unfavourable outcome or avoid an increase in risk for both (BRASIL, 2012, C).

In this context, according to the Ministry of Health's Ordinance No. 570/2000, in accordance with the Prenatal and Birth Humanisation Programme and the Prenatal Care Incentive, it is recommended that at least six prenatal consultations be carried out, one in the first trimester, two in the second and three in the third trimester of pregnancy, with the first consultation preferably taking place by the 4th° month of pregnancy, and one consultation in the puerperium, up to 42 days after delivery (BRASIL, 2000).

Soares and Menezes (2010) argue that insufficient prenatal consultations are strongly related to early neonatal death, reinforcing the need to improve care for pregnant women, care during pregnancy, more assiduous gestational monitoring and early identification of harmful occurrences for the newborn.

Several authors have also confirmed the need for actions that involve not only quantitative care, but also better quality prenatal and birth care, developing more effective strategies for early diagnosis and intervention, training health professionals, greater adherence to the objectives proposed by public maternal-fetal health policies and greater adherence by mothers to appointments, thus preventing various complications, such as low birth weight and prematurity (BRASIL, 2000; BRASIL, 2010 A; BASSO; NEVES; SILVEIRA, 2012; BRASIL, 2012 B; LAMARCA, 2012; ARRUE *et al,* 2013).

However, even with the enormous advances in Brazilian public policies for women's and children's health, many pregnant women still have unsatisfactory antenatal care. Allied to this, many of them still go on pilgrimages to various health services in search of a place at the time of delivery, which can prolong it and subject the child to suffering and complications that could have been avoided, or they come across services that don't use the appropriate and recommended technology for safe and humanised prenatal, labour and birth care (BRASIL, 200; BRASIL, 2010, A).

There is still a dilemma among health professionals when it comes to determining the route of delivery and the ideal time for the birth of the child, especially in high-risk pregnancies, and the decision should be made according to each case, emphasising, however, that high-risk pregnancies are not synonymous with caesarean sections (BRASIL, 2012).

The International Federation of Gynaecology and Obstetrics (FIGO) recommends that the proportion of caesarean sections should not exceed 20% of all deliveries. The World Health Organisation sets a maximum of 15% (SOARES; MENEZES, 2010).

In a study by Cardoso, Albert and Petroianu (2010) on neonatal and maternal morbidity related to the type of delivery, it was concluded that there is greater neonatal morbidity in newborns delivered vaginally compared to newborns delivered by caesarean section and greater maternal morbidity in puerperal women delivered by caesarean section.

Also, according to Silva *et al* (2014), operative delivery in high-risk pregnancies has been considered a relevant procedure for reducing perinatal risks, increasing the survival of newborns, and is indicated, for example, in cases of fetal distress, lack of progress in vaginal labour, pelvic presentation, pre-eclampsia, among others.

In addition to care factors related to prenatal care and childbirth, individual characteristics and unfavourable socio-demographic conditions such as maternal age over 35 or under 15, low schooling, unfavourable environmental conditions, as well as aspects related to previous reproductive history such as preterm births, gestational diabetes and pre-existing medical conditions are also gestational risk factors (BRASIL, 2012).

Azevedo *et al* (2002) and Ximenes and Oliveira (2004) in studies on the influence of maternal age on perinatal conditions show findings that suggest that pregnancy at the extremes of reproductive life is associated with less efficient prenatal care, prematurity, perinatal anoxia and low birth weight.

According to Santos *et al* (2009), teenage pregnancy is often associated with late onset and fewer antenatal appointments, the use of abortifacients in early pregnancy, low schooling, the absence of a partner, low birth weight and prematurity, while in older pregnant women there is a higher incidence of diabetes, pre-eclampsia, premature rupture of membranes and a higher frequency of caesarean section.

In relation to Gestational Age (GA), the World Health Organisation (ICD-10) defines premature babies as those born at less than 37 weeks of GA, establishing the classification of Extreme Premature babies as those born at less than 28 weeks of GA, Very Premature babies as those born between 28 and 31 weeks of GA, Very Premature babies as those born between 32 and 36 weeks and Term babies as those born between 37 and 41 weeks (WORLD HEALTH ORGANISATION, 1995 *apud* FILHO; BARRETO, 2012; BRASIL, 2009).

It should be noted that this condition has been growing in recent years, especially in developed countries, such as the United States, where this demand increased by around 13 per cent between 1991 and 2006. In Brazil, following the global trend, the birth rate of premature newborns rose from 6.5 per cent to around 7.2 per cent between 2004 and 2010 (BRASIL, 2009; FILHO; BARRETO, 2012).

In addition, with regard to the repercussions caused by prematurity, several authors have shown a strong association between this condition and an increase in neonatal and infant morbidity and mortality compared to full-term newborns, with respiratory and metabolic complications, sepsis, intracranial haemorrhage, susceptibility to infections such as necrotising enterocolitis, lower birth weight, longer admission to the NICU, longer use of mechanical ventilation and oxygen therapy, and consequently longer hospital stays, in addition to long-term sequelae and complications (ALVES *et al,* 2012; MACHADO *et al,* 2014).

With regard to birth weight, the term Extreme Low Birth Weight (EBP) is used for newborns weighing < lOOg; Very Low Birth Weight (VLBW) for newborns weighing between 1000 and 1499g; Low Birth Weight (LBW) for newborns weighing between 1500 and 2499g; and Adequate Birth Weight (ADW) for newborns weighing > 2500g according to the classification of birth weight established by the World Health Organisation (ICD-10) (1995) apwí/Filho and Barreto (2012, p.. 404).

As well as prematurity, low birth weight is a risk factor for the development of neonatal complications and morbidities, such as hospital-acquired infections and sepsis, respiratory alterations, jaundice, perinatal anoxia, pulmonary haemorrhage, hypoglycaemia, longer NICU stays and future reintroductions, and the need for mechanical ventilation, suggesting greater priorities in prenatal care in order to minimise this condition, contributing to improving the quality of life of this population and reducing hospital costs with the highly specialised care they need, as well as their sequelae (MALVEIRA *et al,* 2009; LEMOS *etal,* 2010).

Another condition frequently associated with neonatal complications, as reported by authors, is the presence of perinatal anoxia and its relationship with *Apgar* values in the first few minutes of the child's life (FILIZOLA *et al,* 2009; SANTOS; PASQUINI, 2009; SOCIEDADE BRASILEIRA DE PEDIATRIA, 2013).

In 1953, the British anaesthetist Virginia Apgar created the Apgar score to assess the wellbeing of newborns in the delivery room by measuring the physiological conditions and responsiveness of the neonate in terms of heart rate and respiratory effort, muscle tone, reflex irritability and skin colour, assigning scores of 0 to 2 for each item, out of a total of 10 points, and it is still one of the most widely used methods today (SANTOS; PASQUINI, 2009).

Over time, this score has been used to diagnose neonatal asphyxia and, more recently, it has ceased to be an indicator for the start of neonatal resuscitation and is now used to assess the patient's response to the manoeuvres carried out and their effectiveness. It is recommended that the score be documented at the same time as the resuscitation procedures carried out and that it be measured every five minutes up to 20 minutes of life when a value of less than 7 is obtained in the 5th minute° (FILIZOLA *et al,* 2009; SANTOS; PASQUINI, 2009; BRAZILIAN SOCIETY OF PAEDIATRICS, 2013).

However, according to the Ministry of Health's guide on newborn care (2011), neonatal asphyxia can not only be characterised by a condition of metabolic or mixed (metabolic-respiratory) acidemia with a pH of less than 7 in the arterial blood of the umbilical cord and its association with an Apgar score of 0 to 3 for more than 5 minutes, but also by neonatal neurological manifestations such as convulsions, coma or hypotonia and multisystem dysfunction such as multiple organ failure.

However, according to Cunha *et al* (2004), the *Apgar* score may be the only form of general assessment of the neonate in developing countries, where laboratory tests may not be available, indicating when scores are low children who need additional care, even in the absence of laboratory data, and there is a consensus that an Apgar score of 7-10 means a healthy baby who will probably have no future problems, while scores below 7 are a warning sign for special attention.

In a study by Salustiano *et al* (2012) on the conditioning maternal and obstetric factors for low *Apgar scores* in the fifth minute of life in low-risk maternal-infant populations, they concluded that the presence of late intrapartum decelerations (PID II) and a prolonged expulsion period during labour are associated with Apgar scores lower than seven in the fifth minute° , in turn triggering greater respiratory failure at birth, greater need for neonatal ICU and tracheal intubation, as well as the occurrence of hypoxic-ischaemic encephalopathy.

Therefore, based on the above, Carmo *et al* (2004) recognise neonates as a strategic group in terms of child health and morbidity and mortality, and as a parameter for indicating a country's quality of life, level of health and degree of development.

It should also be noted that even though there has been enormous progress in neonatal care over the last century, the World Health Organisation (2001) and the United Nations Children's Fund (2009) estimate that every year, around the world, and especially in developing countries, around four million newborns die before they are 28 days old, with three quarters of these deaths occurring in the first seven days, especially in the first 24 hours after birth, and in most cases these are preventable or treatable deaths (GOMES, 2004; LAWN *et al,* 2005; BRASIL, 2009; BRASIL, 2012).

According to Caderno sobre Situação Mundial da Infância version Brasil 2008, published by UNICEF, when analysed by early neonatal (deaths of children up to 6 days old), late neonatal (deaths of children between 7 and 27 days old) and post-neonatal (deaths of children between 28 and 364 days old) components, it can be seen that newborn care remains very precarious, as approximately 66 per cent of infant deaths occur in the first month of life, 51 per cent of which are early neonatal, mainly related to prematurity, asphyxia during childbirth and infections, but also congenital malformations, low weight and syndromic diseases. (LAWN *et al,* 2005; UNICEF, 2008; ASSIS, 2008; SOARES; MENEZES, 2010; BASSO *et al,* 2012).

Allied to this, Assis (2008) and Tronco *et al* (2010) also state that the precariousness of care and the supply of public services for maternal and newborn health care are related to the main risk factors for neonatal morbidity and mortality, meaning that factors considered avoidable or reducible during pregnancy and childbirth lead to impairment of the newborn and the consequent need for hospitalisation in the NICU.

4.3 Neonatal Intensive Care Units

Neonatal Intensive Care Units (NICUs) are a highly complex therapeutic environment suitable for treating high-risk newborns, offering materials, equipment and diagnostic and therapeutic technology used by a specialised multidisciplinary team that follows specific protocols based on scientific knowledge (KAMADA; ROCHA; BARBEIRA, 2003; ROSA; GAÍVA, 2009).

According to the guidelines established by Ministerial Order No. 930 of 2012, recommended by the Ministry of Health, the NICU can be defined as a hospital service dedicated to the care of critically ill or life-threatening newborns, at any gestational age, who require mechanical ventilation or oxygen support in the acute phase of respiratory failure; those under 30 weeks of gestational age or with a birth weight of less than 1,000 grams; those requiring major surgery or in the immediate post-operative period of small and medium-sized surgeries, as well as parenteral nutrition and other specialised care.

According to the World Health Organisation (WHO), premature newborns are those with a gestational age of less than 37 weeks and a birth weight of 2,500 g or less. They are subdivided into very low birth weight (less than 1,500 grams) and extreme low birth weight (less than 1,000 grams).

Also according to the WHO, babies under 28 weeks are considered extremely premature, having a fragile appearance due to their size and physical characteristics, so they don't have facial features that make it possible for the family to perceive them.

It should also be pointed out that preterm neonates can present a postural pattern in extension, lowered tone, head extension, immaturity of the central nervous system, immaturity of muscles and organs, vital functions with some degree of impairment, absence of reflex automatisms, and a great predisposition to develop clinical complications (DIAS, 2009).

In addition to all the aforementioned alterations, some respiratory disorders are classified as the main causes of hospitalisation in neonatal units. The causes can be pulmonary, anatomical problems compromising the respiratory system, cardiocirculatory, systemic or neuromuscular (SARAIVA 2004).

Respiratory disorders present similar clinical manifestations that reflect the respiratory work of the newborn, are of varying intensity and differ in terms of when they appear (SARAIVA 2004).

In this way, Dias (2009) states that there is an increase in the length of stay of NBs in the NICU, as an early discharge would cause their nervous system, organs and functions to develop in less than ideal conditions, subject to even greater risks and aggressions. The help of a multi-professional team and the affection of their parents are important in overcoming this critical period.

Due to all the peculiarities of the newborn (NB), they are vulnerable to the environment, especially temperature, noise, intense lighting and excessive handling. These conditions are sources of stress for the newborn and the multidisciplinary team, and in NBs they can contribute to increased morbidity. In order to provide adequate care for these babies, it is essential to adapt the environment by minimising the factors that may contribute to their discomfort (CORDEIRO, 2011).

Over the years, with the knowledge of these peculiarities and technological advances, children who until a few years ago were dying in the first few days of life are now surviving (OLIVEIRA, 2008).

This has led to a greater concern on the part of professionals with the patient's clinical condition, often to the detriment of the patient's family, which suffers from the peculiar and premature withdrawal (OLIVEIRA, 2008).

The birth of a high-risk or premature baby is an unforeseen crisis for any family. In the case of the premature newborn, we can consider that the parents are also "premature parents" and face difficulties in dealing with their expectations and reality (SARAIVA, 2004).

Brazil (2010) states that NICUs must meet humanisation requirements for the care and assistance of newborns and their families and have a specialised multidisciplinary team, specific equipment, technology and adequate physical space.

The neonatal intensive care unit is the place that concentrates the main human and material resources needed to provide uninterrupted support for the vital functions of the newborns hospitalised there. There are specialised teams of doctors, nurses and physiotherapists, as well as other health professionals and support staff, backed up by complementary, laboratory and radiological tests, all operating 24 hours a day (CORDEIRO, 2011).

As pointed out by the Brazilian Society of Paediatrics and epidemiological data from the Unified Health System, in recent years there has been an increase in the demand for neonatal intensive care beds and the need to adapt their supply to the current demand of the Brazilian population, with an urgent need for investment, strategic planning, hierarchisation and regionalisation of perinatal care services throughout the country (DATASUS, 2012; SBP, 2012).

Given that prematurity has considerable repercussions on the infant mortality rate, especially in the neonatal period, where the socio-economic and emotional cost of treating these babies is very high, making prematurity a public health problem (DIAS, 2009).

Assis (2008) also points out that the national increase in child health care policies and the increase in neonatal viability has led to the implementation and/or increase in the supply of Neonatal Intensive Care beds in the public sector, mainly in the metropolitan regions of the South and Southeast.

In 2004, according to the WHO, the state of Rio Grande do Sul saw the birth of 153,015 babies, of which 8.5 per cent were premature and 9.3 per cent had low birth weight.

In line with this trend, in 2010 the Ministry of Health established criteria for the expansion and qualification of NICUs throughout the country, especially in the northeastern states and the Legal Amazon, in an attempt to minimise the neonatal fraction of infant mortality and regional inequalities in access to these services, recommending a minimum of four Neonatal Intensive Care beds for every 1,000 live births, and one NICU bed for every three Intermediate Care Unit (ICU) beds (BRASIL, 2010; SBP, 2012).

4.4 Care for newborns in ICUs

Admission to the Neonatal Intensive Care Unit, according to Carmo *et al* (2004), consists of receiving a newborn baby who has difficulties adapting to extrauterine life or pathologies that interfere with their survival in the first month, offering them special care and technologies through a multi-professional team with technical skills and clinical experience, organisation, procedures and protocols aimed at their stability.

Respiratory disorders, low birth weight and prematurity are among the main causes of hospitalisation of neonates in the NICU, while conditions such as neonatal jaundice, infections, congenital malformations and complications arising during labour are also quite common, with more than one causal factor often being associated with hospitalisation (BARBOSA et al, 2007; COELHO; AMARANTE, 2010; BRASIL, 2011; BASSO et al, 2012; DATASUS, 2012; GRANZOTTO et al, 2012; ARRUÉ et al, 2013; TADIELO et al, 2013).

According to the Newborn Health Care Guide, neonatal respiratory disorders can be triggered by the immaturity of the lungs, such as Respiratory Distress Syndrome, disorders caused by complications during the birth process, such as Meconium Aspiration Syndrome, Transient Newborn Tachypnoea and pneumonia, as well as conditions caused by alterations in lung development and growth, such as pulmonary hypoplasia and congenital diaphragmatic hernia, all of which hinder the process of cardiorespiratory adaptation at birth and lead to respiratory failure in the first 72 hours of life, in many cases prolonging hospitalisation and limiting the child's prognosis (BRASIL, 2011).

In addition to these pathologies, the above authors also highlight the existence of high rates of morbidities inherent to prolonged hospitalisation in the NICU and the use of invasive technologies to maintain the stability of the neonate, such as hospital-acquired infections, respiratory, haematological and cardiac disorders, kidney failure, complications from the use of mechanical ventilation, among others.

However, despite the existence of high neonatal morbidity and mortality, the increase in NICUs over the last few decades, as well as the mechanical ventilation techniques applied, therapeutic resources such as the use of exogenous pulmonary surfactant and antenatal corticosteroids, and the improvement in human resources has led to an increase in the survival of children beyond the first 24 hours of birth, a reduction in respiratory disorders and length of hospital stay (THOMPSON; KHOT, 1985; FREDDI et al, 2003; MENEGUEL et al, 2003; MOREIRA, 2004; ASSIS, 2008; BRASIL, 2011; BRASIL, 2012).

Furthermore, according to Lopes (2000), the improved survival of increasingly premature and low birth weight newborns, however, has been accompanied by greater morbidity, especially in relation to chronic lung diseases such as broncho-pulmonary dysplasia (BPD), making these patients dependent on a series of resources for their treatment such as oxygen and/or mechanical ventilation available in NICUs.

With regard to the use of exogenous pulmonary surfactant in premature and low birth weight neonates, it is indicated for prophylactic or therapeutic use in cases of Respiratory Distress Syndrome. In other neonatal lung diseases with surfactant dysfunction, such as Meconium Aspiration Syndrome, pneumonia, pulmonary haemorrhage and Bronchopulmonary Dysplasia, the evidence regarding the effects of such therapy is still poor (JOHNSTON et al, 2008; BRASIL, 2011).

In terms of its benefits, right after administration in the first few hours of life, there is an increase in the functional residual capacity (FRC) of the lungs, thanks to the reduction in surface tension at the alveolar air-liquid interface, the stabilisation of alveoli that are still open and the recruitment of those that are atelectatic, providing more surface area for gas exchange, improving the ventilation-perfusion ratio, reducing the intrapulmonary shunt and, consequently, correcting hypoxaemia and respiratory discomfort (FREDDI et al, 2003; JOHNSTON et al, 2008; BRASIL 2011; MIYOSHI; GUINSBURG, 2008; TEIXEIRA; ALCANTARA, 2010); JOHNSTON et al, 2008; BRASIL, 2011; MIYOSHI; GUINSBURG, 2008; TEIXEIRA; ALCANTARA, 2010).

In the following hours, according to the authors above, a more homogeneous recruitment of alveolar units and an increase in lung compliance are observed, making it possible to reduce invasive ventilatory support. Furthermore, after approximately 6 hours, the need for additional doses should be reassessed.

As an adjunct to the replacement of exogenous pulmonary surfactant, antenatal corticosteroid therapy is indicated for pregnant women at risk of preterm labour between 24 and 34 weeks of gestational age or in other significant clinical situations, such as pre-eclampsia, premature rupture of membranes, premature amniorrexia, placenta previa, intrauterine growth restriction, among others.

Its benefits include the maturation of the newborn's lung function and as a protective factor for the use of mechanical ventilation, oxygen therapy, a reduction in peri-intraventricular hypertension and less need for advanced resuscitation procedures in the delivery room (JOHNSTON et al, 2008; RISSO; NASCIMENTO, 2010; BRASIL, 2011; BITTENCOURT; GRANZOTTO et al, 2012; GAÍVA, 2014; DRUMMOND et al, 2014).

With regard to ventilatory support in the care of newborns in the NICU, Brown and DiBlasi (2011) report that since the creation of the neonatal mechanical ventilator, this resource has been considered an essential tool for the care of newborns with respiratory pathologies, and is still today an integral component in the continuity of neonatal respiratory care, especially in disorders involving increased respiratory effort, inefficient gas exchange, apnoea of prematurity, the need for surfactant replacement therapy, among others.

The main objectives of mechanical ventilation in the neonatal period are to reduce changes in the ventilation/perfusion ratio and improve alveolar ventilation, maintaining normal PACO2; to reduce respiratory work, avoiding muscle fatigue and re-expanding atelectatic areas (CORDEIRO, 2011).

Mechanical lung ventilation attempts to simulate the physiological spontaneous ventilation pattern, using a respiratory rate and tidal volume as close to normal as possible, applying positive pressure to the airways or negative pressure around the chest (CORDEIRO, 2011).

Several authors have discussed the type of ventilatory support for neonates in the NICU, describing that although invasive mechanical ventilation is still the most commonly used form of treatment for lung pathologies, it has also been implicated as a major cause of lung injury, inflammation, risk factor for broncho-pulmonary dysplasia and increased hospital costs, a risk factor for broncho-pulmonary dysplasia and increased hospital costs. Today, there is a greater tendency to use less aggressive ventilation strategies, new ventilation modes, early withdrawal of invasive ventilation or the use of non-invasive ventilation through nasal interfaces, even in increasingly premature and extremely low birth weight neonates (LOPES, 2000; JOHNSTON et al, 2008; BROWN; DIBLASI, 2011; ROBERTS et al, 2011; KIRPALANI et al, 2013; GONÇALVES-FERRI; MARTINEZ, 2013).

Mechanical ventilation should be indicated early, especially in newborns weighing less than 1500g and those who have suffered perinatal asphyxia, to prevent progressive clinical deterioration from hindering the success of ventilotherapy. The main indications are persistent hypoxaemia and/or hypercapnia despite oxygen administration and airway clearance, pulmonary or extrapulmonary clinical conditions in which there is increased respiratory work, with a risk of fatigue and apnoea, altered gas exchange due to a lack of central stimulation or decreased muscle capacity (CORDEIRO, 2011).

In addition, the length of their stay in the unit is prolonged compared to those who do not use mechanical ventilation, and the clinical complications associated with it contribute to this (BARBOSA et al, 2007).

The use of Non-Invasive Ventilation (NIV) in newborns admitted to the NICU offers positive pressure in the airways without the need for oro-tracheal intubation or tracheostomy of the patient, such as CP AP (Continuous positive airways pressure) through a nasal interface, helping to increase transpulmonary pressure, increase capacity and functional residual lung volume, improved lung compliance and gas exchange, prevention of atelectasis, stabilisation of the airways, regularity of respiratory rhythm, among others, as well as reducing the complications of prolonged invasive mechanical ventilation, such as mucosal damage, haemorrhages, tracheal stenosis and infections (LOPES, 2000; JOHNSTON et al, 2008; LEAO et al, 2013).

CHAPTER 5

METHODS

5.1 Ethical standards

The study was carried out in accordance with the precepts of the Guidelines and Regulatory Norms for Research Involving Human Beings imposed by CNS Resolution 466/12, after being approved by the supervisor Professor Dr Aurimery Gomes Chermont and by the Department of Teaching and Research and the Research Ethics Committee of the Santa Casa de Misericórdia Foundation of Pará. With opinion number 1.074.331 on 22/05/2015. And the signing of the Data Use Consent Form (TCUD).

5.2 Characterisation of the study

This is an analytical, comparative and retrospective study of the profile of premature newborns weighing less than or equal to 1,500g admitted to the Intensive Care Units of a single hospital centre in the municipality of Belém - Pará, between January and December 2014, regardless of gender.

The research took place without funding.

5.3 Target population

Newborns weighing less than or equal to 1,500g admitted to neonatal ICUs, regardless of gender, coming from the operating theatre or normal delivery room.

The FSCMPA Neonatal Unit has 60 NICU beds, divided into six units, four on the first floor and two on the seventh floor, each with ten beds.

5.4 Inclusion criteria

Newborns weighing less than or equal to 1,500g, of both sexes, who came from the institution's obstetric ward and required hospitalisation in the neonatal ICUs between January and December 2014, were considered eligible for the study.

5.5-Criteria for exclusion

Medical records with incomplete information according to the data collection form, newborns over 1,500g, or who were born in another hospital, with some kind of congenital malformation and twins.

5. 6-Data collection

After the institution agreed, the medical records were provided by the archive department of the Santa Casa de Misericórdia do Pará Foundation. Data was collected using a form drawn up exclusively for the research, which was filled in according to the information in the patient's medical records, complying with the inclusion criteria. The data was collected by a single researcher in the afternoons on Mondays, Wednesdays and Fridays.

There was no intervention or treatment by the researcher. The following maternal variables were collected: age; origin (own municipality versus others); schooling; parity (primiparous versus non-primiparous); number of prenatal consultations; gestational risk (usual versus high); hospitalisation during pregnancy; use of antenatal corticosteroids and type of delivery (vaginal versus caesarean section). The following newborn variables were assessed: gender, birth weight, gestational age, Apgar score, resuscitation in the delivery room, use of mechanical ventilation and use of surfactant, corticosteroids and number of doses, use of sedation and vasoactive drugs, length of stay in the unit, length of invasive and non-invasive mechanical ventilation, use of drains, use of antibiotics, use of analgesia (pain) and discharge information (APPENDIX A).

Data collection began after the opinion of the teaching and research committee of the Santa Casa de Misericórdia do Pará Foundation with the number 1.074.331 on 22/05/2015, as described in the research schedule, in the month of June and was finalised in July 2015.

5. 7-Statistical analysis

The data was processed in a database created using the Statistical Package for Social Sciences (SPSS) for Windows software version 20.0 (study significance level 5%). The descriptive analysis of the data with absolute numbers and

percentage to obtain the absolute and relative frequencies of the variables analysed, and the prevalence of the outcomes investigated. Mean and standard deviation were calculated for the numerical variables.

In order to check whether the differences between the crossed variables were statistically significant, we used non-parametric tests based on the **sample,** the **variable** and the **type of data** (categorical). The chi-square test of independence was applied apriori to the tables to check whether the differences were statistically significant, but in most of the tables this test was unfeasible because they had a frequency of zero, so in order to solve this problem we used a non-parametric test similar to the chi-square, widely used, known as the G test of independence in the sample of 176 individuals, respecting the basic assumptions for applying these tests. The significance level used in this study was alpha equal to 5% to reject the null hypothesis. All the tests were used with the support of Bioestat software version 5.0.

CHAPTER 6

RESULTS

The study population consisted of 248 medical records of newborns weighing less than or equal to 1,500 grams, admitted to intensive care units between January and December 2014, of which 176 (71%) met the inclusion criteria predetermined in the project and 72 (29%) were excluded according to the defined methodology.

Maternal age ranged from 44 years to 12 years, with an average of 25.06 years.

Mothers aged between 24 and 30 were from the interior of the state, with the municipality of Ananindeua being the most prevalent. Most of the mothers had one or more children.

TABLE 1: Maternal socioeconomic characteristics.

Mother's age group	N	%
10 a 19	47	26,55
20 a 34	106	60,45
Over 35	23	12,99
Origin		
Capital	72	40,90
Inside	105	59,65
Number of pregnancies		
Primipara	73	41,47
No Primipara	103	59,13
Antenatal consultation		
Yes	125	71,03
No	51	28,97
Number of Consultations		
More than 6	31	24,8
Under 6	94	75,2
Prenatal complications		
Yes	97	55,11
No	79	44,83
Prenatal hospitalisation		
Yes	29	16,47
No	147	83,52
Antenatal corticosteroids		
Yes	30	17,04
No	146	82,95
Types of Childbirth		
Caesarean section	93	52,54
Vaginal	83	46,89

Source: Research protocol

With regard to prenatal care, it was noted that most of them had had a consultation, but only incompletely according to the WHO (2012), resulting in a high number of prenatal complications, with urinary tract infection being the most common.

It is interesting to note that antenatal corticosteroids were infrequent and the type of birth was similar.

Table 2 and 3 show the data of the newborns admitted to the ICUs

TABLE 2: Characteristics of newborns admitted to ICUs.

Sex	N	%
Male	97	55,11
Female	79	44,88
Gestational age		
Less than 28	40	22,72
28 a 31	83	47,15
32 a 36	52	29,54
37 a 41	1	0,56
Over 41	0	
Weight		
496 a 696	37	21
697 a 896	41	23,2
897 a 1096	40	22,7
1097 a 1296	32	18
1297 a 1500	26	14,7
Resuscitation in the labour room		
Yes	100	56,81
No	76	43,18
Surfactant		
Yes	149	84,65
No	27	15,34
Vasoactive drugs		
Yes	157	89,20
No	19	10,79
VAD scheme		
Dopamine+dobutamine	85	54,14
Adrenaline+Dopamine+Dobutamine	62	38,85
Dopamine	6	3,82
Adrenaline+Dopamine	3	1,91
Adrenaline	2	1,27
Sedative Analgesic		
Midazolan+F entanil	67	56,30
Midazolan	26	21,36
Fentanyl	19	15,45
Ventilator Resource		
Mechanical ventilation	162	92,04
Non-invasive ventilation	9	5,11
Oxihood	5	2,82

Source: Research protocol

Gestational age ranged from 20 to 41 weeks, with an average of 29.85.

The predominant gestational age was 28 to 31 weeks, and the weight ranged from 496g to 1485g with an average of 955g.

The Apgar score after 5 minutes was 7.36 on average, however, most of the newborns underwent some kind of resuscitation in the delivery room. With regard to the resources used, many were given surfactant while still in the delivery room, as well as vasoactive drugs, with dopamine and dobutamine being the most common combination.

Sedation and analgesia were indicated in 67 (56.30%) of the NBs, and the most frequent combination was midazolam with fentanyl. The minimum time sedation/analgesia was used was 24 hours and the maximum was 69 days, with an average of 8.73 days.

However, the most commonly used ventilatory support was mechanical ventilation via tracheal tube in SIMV-TCLP with 162 (92.04%). The maximum duration of mechanical ventilation was 69 days and the minimum was just one day (average of 9.90 days). Of the total number of NBs, 38 (21.5%) used non-invasive ventilation, with a maximum of 45 days and a minimum of one day and an average of 9.19 days. Only four (2.27%) newborns required a tracheostomy.

Five babies (2.84%) used drains, of which the thoracic drain was the most frequently used for hypertensive pneumothorax.

TABLE 3: Newborn hospitalisation data.

ICU time	N	%
Up to 7	98	55,68
8 a 14	24	13,63
15a21	23	13,06
22 a 28	12	6,81
>a29	19	10,79
Complications		
Yes	171	97,15
No	5	2,84
Main complications		
Hypovolaemic Shock	64	36,36
Sepsis	61	34,65
Pulmonary haemorrhage	30	17,04
Pneumonia	22	12,5%
Infection		
Yes	106	60,22
No	70	39,78
Culture		
ICS	51	48,11
Lungs	45	42,45
Urine	1	0,94
LCR	1	0,94
Agents		
Klebsiella *sp*	28	26,41
Candida *sp*	22	20,75
Acinetobacter *sp*	23	21,69
Staphylococcus *sp*	13	12,26
Antibiotic generation		
1st generation	124	70,45
2° generation	13	7,38
3° generation	21	11,93
4° generation	18	10,22

Source: Research protocol

TABLE 3 shows that the minimum ICU stay was just one day and the maximum was 145 days, with an average length of stay of 13.15 days.

Table 4, 5 and 6 show the discharge data and the correlations with neonatal death.

TABLE 4: Type of discharge and diagnosis in the NB's OR

Types of discharge	N	%

Discharge from the unit	33	18,75
Transfer	1	0,0005
Death	142	80,68
Death bulletin		
Septic Shock	42	29,57
Pulmonary haemorrhage	58	40,84
Obstructive Shock	3	2,11
Sepsis	4	2,81
Extreme prematurity	23	16,19
Respiratory failure	8	5,63

Source: Research protocol

TABLE 5: Frequency of neonatal deaths according to variables about the length of stay in hospital.

	Death						
	Yes		No		Total		
Variables	n	%	n	%	n	%	p
Birth weight range							*0,001*
496 alOOg	92	64,8	11	32,4	103	58,5	
1001 to 1500g	**50**	35,2	23	67,6	73	41,5	
Length of stay in the ICU							*0,000*
Up to 7 days	94	66,2	4	11,8	98	55,7	
More than 7 days	48	33,8	30	88,2	78	44,3	
Mechanical ventilation time							0,187
Up to 10 days	103	72,5	11	57,9	114	70,8	
More than 10 days	39	27,5	8	42,1	47	29,2	
Not realised	84	59,2	19	55,9	103	58,5	
Complete prenatal care							0,620
Yes	26	18,3	5	14,7	31	17,6	
No	116	81,7	29	85,3	145	82,4	
Corticosteroids							0,541
Yes	23	16,2	7	20,6	30	17,0	
No	119	83,8	27	79,4	146	83,0	
Surfactant							*0,000*
Yes	128	90,1	21	61,8	149	84,7	
No	14	9,9	13	38,2	27	15,3	
Sedation							0,074
Midazolan+F ent	54	38,0	13	38,2	67	38,1	
Midazolan	25	17,6	1	2,9	26	14,8	
Not realised	63	44,4	20	58,8	83	47,2	
Complications							*0,001*
Shock Hyp. + Sepsis	142	100,0	30	88,2	172	97,7	
H. Pulmonary + PNM	0	0,0	4	11,8	4	2,3	
Infection							0,564
Yes	87	61,3	19	55,9	106	60,2	
No	55	38,7	15	44,1	70	39,8	
Infectious agent							0,581
Fungi	19	13,4	3	8,8	22	12,5	
Gram-negative	39	27,5	12	35,3	51	29,0	
No information	84	59,2	19	55,9	103	58,5	
Total	**142**	**100,0**	34	**100,0**	**176**	**100,0**	-

p: probability calculated using the Chi-squared test.

Table 4 shows that of the 176 neonates, 142 (80%) died. When weight was compared with the outcome of the babies, it was observed that the lower the weight, the greater the likelihood of death. The shorter the length of stay also showed strong significance in relation to death.

Other variables proved to be significant in relation to the death outcome. The use of surfactant in the delivery room was one of these. As well as complications in the NICU such as hypovolaemic shock associated with sepsis, the prognosis was unfavourable for neonates. When correlating other variables, there was no statistical significance in relation to the type of discharge.

Table 6 analyses the logistic regression for death, showing that the lower the weight (<1000g) and the shorter the length of stay, the greater the chance of death (3.85/ 0.07). A similar result was found for ventilation time > 10 days (6.74). The other variables showed lower odds ratios.

TABLE 6: Logistic regression analysis of death according to characterisation variables.

Variable	Crude OR (CI95 .)%	P	Adjusted OR (IC95)%	P
Birth weight range		*0,001*		0,171
496 alOOg	3,85 (1,73;8,55)		2,61 (0,66; 10,32)	
1001al500g	1		1	
Length of stay in the ICU		*0,000*		*0,000*
Up to 7 days	0,07 (0,02;0,21)		0.01 (0.00;0.ll)	
More than 7 days	1		1	
Mechanical ventilation time		0,312		*0,026*
More than 10 days	0,52 (0,19; 1,39)		6,74 (1,25;36,31)	
Up to 10 days	1		1	
Complete prenatal care		0,622		0,892
Yes	0,77 (0,27;2,18)		0,89 (0,17;4,57)	
No	1		1	
Corticosteroids		0,543		0,881
Yes	0,75 (0,29; 1,92)		0,87 (0,15;5,07)	
No	1		1	
Surfactant		*0,000*		0,261
Yes	5,66 (2,33;13,75)		0,36 (0,06;2,15)	
No	1		1	
Sedation				
Midazolan+F ent	1,32 (0,60;2,90)	0,492	0,20 (0,04;0,91)	*0,037*
Midazolan	7,94 (1,00;62,71)	*0,050*	1,63 (0,13;20,56)	0,704
Not realised	1		1	
Infection		0,566		*0,041*
Yes	1,25 (0,58;2,67)		8,31 (1,10;62,95)	
No	1		1	
Infectious agent				
Fungi	1,43 (0,38;5,36)	0,593	0,55 (0,07;4,28)	0,565
Gram-negative	0,74 (0,32; 1,67)	0,461	0,30 (0,04;2,14)	0,230
No information	1		1	

Crude OR: odds ratio (OR) with unadjusted variables - bivariate analysis. **$CI_{95\%}$** : 95% confidence interval. p:0.079 chi-square test probability. **Adjusted OR:** OR with variables adjusted for each other - multiple analysis.

CHAPTER 7

DISCUSSION

7.1 Maternal descriptive characteristics.

The study of 176 newborns weighing less than or equal to 1,500g showed a predominance of mothers in the same age bracket as several studies (GALVÃO, 2015), i.e. between 20 and 30 years old.

This finding is in line with Franco and Moutinho's (2013) study on the epidemiological assessment of the mother-child binomial carried out at the FSCMPA, concluding that most of the parturients treated at the maternity hospital were between 18 and 24 years old.

On this subject, several authors point to the age group between 20 and 25 as the best maternal age from a reproductive point of view, a period considered to have the lowest perinatal risk.

Thus, at the extremes of maternal reproductive life, complications often occur, which can lead, among other things, to preterm labour and low birth weight, and consequently a greater need for the neonate to be hospitalised in a neonatal ICU.

Adolescence in itself is not a risk factor for pregnancy, however, there is a greater possibility of psychosocial risk and emotional immaturity, with various repercussions on the pregnant woman's life, which may translate into her not adhering to the recommendations made during prenatal care (AZEVEDO *et al,* 2002; BRASIL, 2010, A; RIBEIRO, 2011; BUSTAMANTE 2014; COSTA *et al,* 2014).

The lack of financial resources in the care networks, and the precarious health system at all levels, means that care intensifies in hospitals in the capitals of all Brazilian states. Galvão *et al* in 2010 cited in their study of a NICU in Ceará that more than 80% of mothers came from the interior of the state, corroborating our study which found 59%.

Lamarca (2012) draws attention to the precariousness of prenatal and birth care services in the north of the country, with huge discrepancies in relation to the south and southeast, and the heterogeneous spatial distribution of health services, which therefore means fewer prenatal consultations and probably more unfavourable pregnancy outcomes, as well as diagnosing serious social inequality.

It is known that the internalisation of municipalities such as Abaetetuba, Parauapebas, Marabá, Santarém and Tucuruí, although they have NICUs, their number is below ten beds, which does not meet the population's needs.

The Brazilian Society of Paediatrics (2012) reported that the number of neonatal ICU beds per 1,000 live births compared to the estimate of their real need showed great differences in the distribution of neonatal ICU beds between Brazilian regions, with a great shortage of public neonatal beds in the North and Northeast regions, reflecting, in addition to the inadequacy of the quantity compared to the need, a precariousness of the basic perinatal care network in these places.

It should also be noted that the predominance of pregnant women/newborns coming from municipalities in the interior of the state reflects the fact that the FSCMPará is the only maternal and child reference hospital for teaching and assistance to the SUS in the municipality of Belém, thus meeting the demand from patients coming from other municipalities.

As for parity, this study showed that almost 60 per cent of pregnant women were multiparous. Ribeiro, in his research, tried to associate the number of pregnancies as a risk factor for newborns admitted to the NICU in Recife, and found no statistical significance in this category, emphasising the opposite, that mothers with more than one child would have more experience in pregnancies, not causing possible pathologies triggered by stress. (RIBEIRO, 2009).

The study showed that almost 71 per cent of mothers had prenatal care. However, 75 per cent of these were incomplete. Similar data was found by Costa *et al* (2014) in a NICU in Fortaleza/CE in relation to prenatal care, where 7 (6.3%) of 111 mothers had not had any appointments, 66 (59.5%) had one to five appointments and 38 (34.2%) had six to 12 appointments.

Unlike Silveira *et al* (2012), who associated prenatal care with neonatal morbidity in a NICU in a public hospital in the southern region of Brazil, who found that 87% of mothers had more than six complete prenatal consultations. As well as the studies by Pieszak *et al* (2013) in a NICU in Rio Grande do Sul, 79.8 per cent of mothers had complete prenatal care.

It is assumed from the above data, as well as Lamarca (2012) and a national study on the proportion of live births with seven or more antenatal care visits per year, according to region and maternal schooling, that there is a large inter-regional difference in access to antenatal care services in Brazil, given that in 2010, the South region, for example, had 75.3 per cent of live births with seven or more antenatal care visits, while in the North this proportion was 36.8 per cent (Northeast region 45.3 per cent; Central region 67.2 per cent; Southeast region 72.7 per cent); Centre-West region 67.2%; Southeast region 72.7%), contributing to higher risks of complications during childbirth as well as maternal hospitalisations (BRASIL, 2012, B; LAMARCA, 2012).

In this context, the number of prenatal consultations is a protective factor in relation to maternal and child risks and problems. In addition to the number of consultations, the quality of care services during this period should also be valued, with the use of the necessary equipment and instruments, the training of the health team, and the early start of consultations (BRASIL, 2000; BRASIL, 2010 A; BASSO; NEVES; SILVEIRA, 2012; BRASIL, 2012 B; LAMARCA, 2012; ARRUE *et al,* 2013).

The use of corticosteroids was minimised, as around 82% of the mothers did not receive them. Even so, of the 30 (17%) NBs who benefited, only seven (23%) were discharged and of the 23 (76.6%) who died, early mortality occurred in 16 (69.5%) of them.

These results differ from those of Drummond *et al* (2014), who found that in a NICU at a University Hospital in Niterói/RJ, 82.7% of newborns with a gestational age of up to 34 weeks and a weight of up to 1,500g were given antenatal corticosteroids by their mothers. Like Granzotto *et al* (2012) and Risso *et al* (2010), who in their studies also reported the use of antenatal corticosteroid therapy in mothers of neonates under 34 weeks. Perhaps this was due to incomplete prenatal care.

On this subject, Bittencourt and Gaíva (2014), in a study on early neonatal mortality related to clinical interventions in the delivery room and NICU in Cuiabá/MT, argue that interventions to minimise respiratory failure and neonatal lung damage should begin in the gestational period, administering antenatal corticosteroids in a timely manner to pregnant women at risk of preterm labour, providing the neonate with better birth conditions, less need for aggressive interventions, better respiratory performance, reduced use of exogenous surfactant in the delivery room and less time on mechanical ventilation.

In addition, the aforementioned authors also recognise that despite the proven benefits of antenatal corticosteroids in the prophylaxis of pulmonary complications, as a protective factor for mechanical ventilation and oxygen therapy for premature newborns, as well as the reduced need for advanced resuscitation procedures in the delivery room, their use is still restricted to a small number of pregnant women who should use them (RISSO; NASCIMENTO, 2010; GRANZOTTO *et al,* 2012; BITTENCOURT; GAÍVA, 2014; DRUMMOND *et al,* 2014).

As for the type of delivery, there was no difference between caesarean and vaginal deliveries (52.54% X 46.89%). Similarly, Lages *et al* (2014) found higher percentages of caesarean deliveries in a NICU of a public maternity hospital in Piauí, with 55.1% of caesarean deliveries. Risso and Nascimento (2010) in the NICU of a university hospital in Taubaté/SP between 2005 and 2007 with 57.20 per cent of caesarean deliveries, Benites and Nunes (2006) in the NICU of Campo Grande/MS in 2002, with 58.2 per cent of caesarean sections, Bustamante *et al* (2014) in the NICU of Minas Gerais with caesarean sections in 60,3% of mothers, Tragante (2009) in the NICU of the Hospital das

Clínicas of the Faculty of Medicine of the University of São Paulo with 59.2% caesarean sections and Pieszak *et al* (2013) in the NICU of a teaching hospital in Rio Grande do Sul between 2002 and 2006, with 76% of caesarean deliveries.

The number of caesarean deliveries in this study can be explained by the fact that the FSCMPA, like the other hospitals mentioned above, is a teaching hospital and a state reference in high-risk prenatal, labour and birth care, with an intense and continuous flow of pregnant women from all over the state, with care provided by spontaneous demand or referrals. Therefore, it is assumed that the small difference of 52% vs. 46% may suggest poor basic prenatal care as well as poor quality, often putting these puerperal women into premature labour that could not be prevented.

Reinforcing this idea, Barbosa, Chaves and Campos (2007) in a study on the characterisation of newborns on mechanical ventilation in a public Neonatal Unit in the municipality of Fortaleza/CE found that of the 42 newborns studied, 23 (54.8%) were born by caesarean section, while 15 (35.6%) were born vaginally, as well as one (2.4%) by pelvic delivery and three (7.2%) had no information in their medical records.

With regard to this issue, several studies have pointed to an increase in maternal and neonatal morbidity and mortality rates associated with caesarean section when compared to vaginal delivery. However, operative delivery in high-risk pregnancies has been considered a relevant procedure for reducing perinatal risks and increasing newborn survival. It is indicated, for example, in cases of fetal distress, lack of progress in vaginal labour, pelvic presentation, pre-eclampsia and oligoamnio (SILVA *et al,* 2014).

7.2 Characteristics of newborns admitted to ICUs.

In this study, although 55 per cent of NBs were male, there was no statistical difference between the sexes. Similar results to those found in this study have been found in the literature, with a slight predominance of males over females in NICUs, as in the work by Lages *et al* (2014) with 376 newborns in a NICU in Piauí, of which 207 (55.1%) were male, Arrué *et al* (2013) with 302 newborns admitted to the NICU of a University Hospital in Santa Maria/RS, with 192 (58%) of these being male, Risso and Nascimento (2010) with information on 491 newborns admitted to the Taubaté/SP NICU between 2005 and 2007, with 272 (55.40%) being male and Ponciano *et al* (2008) with 411 newborns admitted to the NICU of a public hospital in João Pessoa/PB, with 225 (54.74%) being male.

Few studies have found higher numbers of females in NICU admissions, such as Bustamante *et al* (2014) with 35 (51.5%) of 68 female NBs in a NICU in the interior of Minas Gerais. However, male babies had a higher death rate (21.2%) in this NICU compared to females (14.3%).

This can be explained by the study by Peacock *et al* (2012), which showed a strong association between preterm male neonates and a greater risk of morbidity and mortality compared to females, as well as an association with lower gestational ages at birth, longer hospital stays, greater oxygen dependency, greater pulmonary haemorrhage and the use of postnatal steroids, lower *Apgar* scores at birth, among others, suggesting that female neonates have more advanced lung maturity in the last months of pregnancy, in addition to the protective oestrogenic factor for the immune system and a more efficient response to maternal antenatal corticosteroids and exogenous pulmonary surfactant compared to males with greater exposure to androgenic hormones inhibiting their production and effectiveness.

For the most frequent gestational age variable, the study found a range of 28 to 31 weeks - 47.15%. High percentages of prematurity, *albeit* to a lesser extent than that found in this study, were also obtained in the work of Granzotto *et al* (2012) in three consecutive years in a NICU in Pelotas/RS, with percentages of premature NBs of 71.1%, 72.8% and 75.2%,1%, 72.8% and 75.2%, Basso, Neves and Silveira (2012) in the neonatal ICU of a teaching hospital in Santa Maria/RS with 65% of premature newborns, Bustamante *et al* (2014) in the Itajubá/MG NICU with 70.58% of premature babies, Silva *et al* (2014) in 34 High Risk Neonatal Units that are part of the North-Northeast Perinatal Health Network in 9 states in the Northeast region of Brazil with 78.9% of premature babies, Benites and Nunes (2006) in a NICU in Campo Grande/MS in 2002 with 64.1% of premature babies, Lages *et al* (2014) in the NICU of a public maternity hospital in the state of Piauí with 85.4% of premature babies and 66.4% according to data from the NICU of the Sofia Feldman Maternal and Child Care Reference Hospital in Belo Horizonte/MG in the first half of 2014.

The lowest percentage of prematurity was found in a study by Tragante (2009) in the Neonatal Intensive Care Unit of the Hospital das Clínicas of the University of São Paulo Medical School, in which 39.4% of the newborns admitted had a gestational age between 26 and 28 weeks, which corresponded to only 40 (22.72%) in the present study.

With regard to the repercussions caused by prematurity, Machado *et al* (2014) in a systematic review on the subject revealed a strong association between this condition and an increase in neonatal and infant morbidity and mortality compared to full-term NBs, the main complications being respiratory, metabolic, infectious, intracranial haemorrhage, necrotising enterocolitis, increased admission to the Neonatal Intensive Care Unit and prolonged hospital stays, as well as long-term sequelae and complications.

In addition, several studies on the characterisation of the morbidity and mortality of NBs in

NICUs, such as Arrué *et al* (2013) in the NICU of a University Hospital in Santa Maria/RS, found prematurity and its complications during childbirth to be the main risk factors for neonatal death in these units, when compared to other perinatal factors.

Like Kassar *et al* (2013) in a study on risk factors for neonatal mortality, they identified low birth weight, associated with inadequate prenatal care and the admission of the NB to the ICU, as strong contributors. Figueiró-Filho *et al* (2014) found similar studies in which very low birth weight NBs admitted to the neonatal ICU of a university hospital in Campo Grande, Mato Grosso do Sul showed a significant association with the occurrence of metabolic, neurological and infectious comorbidities, a longer period of hospitalisation and early neonatal death.

In this study, the *Apgar score,* unlike most studies, was seven in the fifth minute (RISSO; NASCIMENTO, 2010; GRANZOTTO *et al,* 2012; BITTENCOURT; GAÍVA, 2014; DRUMMOND *et al,* 2014). However, this positive result did not prevent the need for resuscitation in the delivery room, which occurred in 100 (56.81%) babies and of these the majority 81 (46%) were resuscitated with a bag-valve-mask using 100% oxygen. However, in the NICU 162 (92%) babies arrived intubated with a 100% bag-valve-mask. In this context, the evidence shows that such use of a high concentration of oxygen could be minimised with the use of the Babypuff, maintaining a low PIP and PEEP, avoiding barotrauma and oxidative stress, which is harmful to premature lungs. (SÁ, 2010; Guidelines 2016 of the Brazilian Paediatric Society 26 January 2016)

With regard to the Apgar score and resuscitation in the delivery room, the work by Granzotto *et al* (2012) in the NICU of a teaching hospital in Pelotas/RS revealed *Apgar scores of* less than seven in the fifth week, which is different from the results of this study. Similar data was found by Risso and Nascimento (2010) in the NICU of a university hospital in Taubaté/SP between 2005 and 2007. They analysed 183 (38.28%) of 478 NBs with *Apgar* scores lower than seven at 5° minutes.

Like the publication by Salustiano *et al* (2012) on obstetric and maternal factors conditioning low *Apgar* scores in the fifth minute of life in low-risk maternal-infant populations, they conclude that the presence of late intrapartum decelerations (PID II) and a prolonged expulsion period during labour are associated with *Apgar scores* below seven in the fifth minute°, which is an indication of perinatal anoxia, in turn triggering greater respiratory failure at birth, greater need for NICU and tracheal intubation, as well as the occurrence of hypoxic-ischaemic encephalopathy, reinforcing the importance of adequate maternal and child care during this period.

The use of pulmonary surfactant in the delivery room was found in 149 (84.65%) of the NBs, obviously due to their gestational age. According to Polin et al (2016) the use of surfactant can sharply reduce the morbidity and mortality rate, but the timing of use must be considered, requiring observation of the babies and thus the use of exogenous surfactant, because when Polin analysed the two moments of use, the first right in the delivery room (Prophylaxis) and the second inside the intensive care units (Rescue) in the meta-analysis his results when applied routinely prophylactically (within 2 hours) versus Rescue concluded that the risks of mortality (RR 0.84; 95% Cl 0.74-0.95), auto PEEP (RR 0.61; 95% CI 0.48-0.78), bronchopulmonary dysplasia (RR 0.69; 95% CI 0.55-0.86), and chronic lung disease or death (RR 0.83; 95% CI 0.75-0.91).

It is interesting to remember that the same Polin found that NBs born before 32 weeks and whose mothers received antenatal corticosteroids and surfactant in the form of rescue, the aforementioned subgroup showed a significant reduction in mortality, severity of respiratory distress, and auto PEEP when compared to the subgroup that did not receive it. These findings corroborate evidence from animal models (Polin, 2016).

The articles by Teixeira and Alcântara (2010) in a NICU in Manaus/AM and by Argondizzo (2013) in a NICU in Pelotas/RS revealed that in the first study, 34 (30.91%) of the 110 premature NBs received pulmonary surfactant while 76 (69.09%) did not, with extreme and very low birth weight premature neonates receiving more surfactant than moderate ones. In the second study, 52 (48.6%) of the NBs admitted were given surfactant, with use decreasing as gestational age increased.

According to the Ministry of Health's Guide to High-Risk Pregnancy (Brazil, 2011, B), the use of exogenous pulmonary surfactant in the delivery room reduces the risk of neonatal death by stabilising the alveoli, increasing the functional residual capacity of the lung, improving the ventilation-perfusion ratio and, consequently, correcting hypoxaemia. It is used in association with other strategies, such as antenatal corticotherapy, as adjunct therapies in the treatment of Acute Respiratory Failure.

Bittencourt and Gaíva (2014), in a study on early neonatal mortality related to clinical interventions in the delivery room and NICU in Cuiabá/MT, pointed out that the use of exogenous pulmonary surfactant did not show a statistically significant association with early neonatal mortality; however, among the neonates who died in the first week of life, the majority did not use surfactant, unlike our results.

The use of pharmacological management reported by Silveira et al (2010) corroborates the assistance found in the present study. The use of vasoactive drugs in neonates with haemodynamic shock, after volumetric therapy, has been much debated as to which regimen should be used. The same study found that the use of dobutamine in association with noradrenaline had an early reversal effect on haemodynamic instability. This is related to an improved prognosis and cardiac resuscitation rate.

In agreement with this research, Silva *et al* (2015) found statistical significance in their cohort study on neonatal sepsis in NBs under 1500g, with regard to the relationship between vasoactive drugs and length of stay in the NICU, thus demonstrating that drug management directly interferes with the prognosis of these patients.

Matos *et al* (2015) were concerned with describing the use of sedatives and analgesics in newborns. Their findings were similar to the present study, reporting that the use of midazolam and fentanyl to relieve neonatal pain and stress, triggered by various factors such as: prolonged mechanical ventilation, inadequate nutrition, episodes of falling oxygen saturation, intense lighting, constant noise, multiple procedures, describing that use should be individualised.

Likewise, Bergman *et al*'s (2009) retrospective review of records of children treated in intensive care with prolonged midazolam infusion revealed neurological sequelae in 11.1% of children who received prolonged midazolam infusion. In all these cases, the effects were transient, although no follow-up has been reported on these NBs.

Harter *et al* (2009) and Van Straaten *et al* (2008) reported a significant decrease in blood flow velocity in the middle cerebral artery in preterm NBs with the administration of a single bolus of midazolam. This effect lasted one hour and was directly related to a drop in blood pressure. Thus, it seems that the neurological effects of midazolam may be primarily related to transient cerebral hypoperfusion.

Waisman *et al* (2008) described marked myoclonic spasms, reminiscent of clonic convulsions, within five minutes of receiving a slow bolus of 0.lmg/kg midazolam for sedation. Gestational ages were 24, 25 and 26 weeks, with an average weight of 67 Ig. The drug was administered at 28, 32 and two days, respectively. The abnormal movement improved within 5-10 minutes. These findings are probably due to the changes described in the haemodynamics of cerebral blood flow

The mechanism of hypotension related to midazolam was thought to be due to vasodilation related to extravascular prostanoid and calcium levels (Modanlou *et al,* 2008). More recently, Ahmad et al (2008), in an experimental study, showed that after an attack dose of midazolam there was a change in systemic prostanoid production and in the sagittal sinus. These changes may reflect a decrease in cerebral perfusion and metabolism during midazolam infusion.

Burtin *et al* (2007) reported arterial hypotension in six newborns with hyaline membrane disease after the use of midazolam loading dose (five cases) or during concomitant administration with fentanyl (five cases). Therefore, the loading dose of midazolam in premature NBs, as well as the combination with fentanyl, should be used with great care, especially in premature NBs or neonates with unstable blood pressure. Jacqz-Aigrain *et al* (2009) reported hypotension in four babies receiving continuous infusion (after an attack) of midazolam, three of whom received fentanyl.

When the ventilation resources used in the study were evaluated, mechanical ventilation was present in the majority of babies, 162 (92.04%), non-invasive ventilation in nine (5.11%) and circulating oxygen therapy in five (2.82%).

Risso and Nascimento (2010), who collected information from 485 low birth weight NBs admitted to the NICU in Taubaté, São Paulo, in relation to the use or not of mechanical ventilation, found that 424 (87.42%) of them did not use it, compared to 61 (12.58%) babies who did.

These authors also obtained information on 479 NBs who did or did not use NIV (called positive pressure ventilation by the authors) admitted to this same NICU, finding that 347 (72.44%) did not use it compared to only 132 (27.56%). Similarly, information on the 493 NBs who did or did not receive FiO2 above 21% (or oxygen therapy, as the authors also call it) was present in 288 (58.42%) compared to 205 (41.58%).

Granzotto, Fonseca and Lindemann (2012) in a NICU in Pelotas/RS in 2006 showed that 80.2% of the 172 neonates admitted received circulating oxygen, and 79.9% received CP AP.

For them, in the period between 2008 and 2010, the number of NBs ventilated with positive pressure (also described as mechanical ventilation) increased from 39.7 per cent in 2008 to 42.1 per cent in 2009 and 43.7 per cent in 2010.

The data from the study by Piccoli *et al* (2012) on the clinical profile of very low birth weight neonates admitted to a NICU in Porto Alegre/RS in 2009 was more similar to the data from the present study, where 97 (61.7%) of the 153 neonates analysed required invasive ventilatory support, while 26 (16.5%) did not.

In the results of Teixeira and Alcântara (2010), who analysed the use of surfactant, ventilatory support, length of stay and number of deaths in premature infants of different gestational ages in the NICU of Manaus/AM in 2009, they found that 45 (40.91%) of the 110 neonates received mechanical ventilation, while 65 (59.09%) did not. Regarding the use of nasal AP CP and *oxihood,* 68 (61.82%) and 31 (28.18%) neonates used them respectively.

Several authors have discussed ventilatory support for neonates in the NICU, describing that although invasive mechanical ventilation is still the most commonly used form of treatment for lung pathologies, it has also been implicated as a major cause of lung injury, inflammation, risk factor for bronchopulmonary dysplasia and increased hospital costs, a risk factor for bronchopulmonary dysplasia and an increase in hospital costs. There has been a worldwide trend towards the use of less aggressive ventilation strategies, new ventilation models, early withdrawal of invasive ventilation or the use of non-invasive ventilation via nasal interfaces, even in increasingly premature and extremely low birth weight neonates (LOPES, 2000; JOHNSTON *et al,* 2008; BROWN; DIBLASI, 2011; ROBERTS *et al,* 2011; KIRPALANI *et al,* 2013; GONÇALVES- FERRI; MARTINEZ, 2013).

In addition, Gonçalves-Ferri and Martinez (2013), in a study of nasal CPAP used prophylactically in extremely low birth weight premature infants at a university hospital in São José dos Campos/SP, point out that in order for new non-invasive ventilation measures to be used successfully in populations with low resources and unfavourable neonatal conditions, there is a need for greater and better care not only for the neonate in the peri- and post-natal period, but also for prenatal monitoring, with protective strategies such as antenatal corticosteroids and the prevention of maternal and child risk factors.

With regard to length of stay in this study, we found that the majority of NBs stayed in the NICU for up to seven days, 98 (55.68%), and 78 (44.7%) had a longer stay in the units.

The studies found in the literature showed an average length of stay close to that found in this study, such as Basso, Neves and Silveira (2012) in a NICU in Rio Grande do Sul in 2006, with a length of stay for low birth weight neonates ranging from 1 to 160 days, with an average length of stay of 19.6 days and Bustamante *et al* (2014) in a NICU in Minas Gerais, between 2012 and 2013, with an average of 21 days, showing a considerable discrepancy from our results of an average of 13.15 days.

However, other results were found in the study by Granzotto, Fonseca and Lindemann (2012) in the NICU of Pelotas, RS, in 2006, with an average length of stay of 17 days; Benites and Nunes (2006) in the NICU of Campo Grande, MS, in 2002, with an average length of stay of 11.6 days; and an average of 15 days, 15 days and 13 days in the NICU of the Sofia Feldman Hospital in Belo Horizonte, MG, for the years 2012, 2013 and the first half of 2014, respectively. This corroborates our findings.

In an article by the Brazilian Society of Paediatrics (2012) on the relationship between the number of neonatal ICU beds per 1,000 live births and the estimated need for neonatal ICU beds in Brazil, it is pointed out that information on the length of stay of high-risk newborns in NICUs is scarce and varies greatly from one hospital to another, depending on the characteristics of the population being cared for, the criteria for admission to the NICU and the quality of care provided.

Therefore, this data may suggest that the average number of days spent in hospital tends to be characterised according to the severity of the people being cared for, suggesting higher average lengths of stay in more complex NICUs located in high-risk hospitals of reference for mothers and children.

This study showed that the main complications during hospitalisation occurred in almost all of the study subjects 171 (97.15%), and of these hypovolaemic shock occurred in 64 (36.36%) followed by sepsis 61 (34.65%) followed by pulmonary haemorrhage 30 (17.04%) demonstrating that the same ventilatory, nutritional and medication strategy needs to be differentiated according to the gestational age and weight of the NBs in the study.

The complications and reasons for hospitalisation were diverse, similar results to this study were found in the work of Arrué *et al* (2013) in a NICU in Santa Maria/RS with Prematurity in 172 (57%) of 302 newborns, followed by respiratory distress in 172 (57%) and hypovolaemic shock in 29 (10%) and Piesak *et al* (2013) in a NICU also in Santa Maria/RS between 2002 and 2006 with prematurity in 888 (54.5%) of 1628 neonates, respiratory causes in 881 (54.1%) and low weight in 288 (17.7%) as the main reasons, showing an association of complications at the time of hospitalisation.

As in the studies by Lages *et al* (2014) in a NICU in Teresina, PI, where the main complications during hospitalisation were respiratory problems (57.2%), followed by haemodynamic shocks (34.0%) and some type of infection (4.5%), as well as Tadielo *et al* (2013) in a NICU in a teaching hospital in southern Brazil with respiratory distress (50.5%) and neonatal infection (12.8%), Ponciano *et al* (2008) in a NICU in João Pessoa/PB between 2004 and 2008 with Cardiopulmonary Diseases (38.93%) followed by prematurity (23,60%) and Malformative Syndromes (19.70%), Costa *et al* (2014) in a Fortaleza/CE NICU with haemodynamic shocks (55.5%) followed by risk of intrapartum infection (41.8%) and respiratory distress (35.5%), Basso, Neves and Silveira (2012) in a Rio Grande do Sul NICU with respiratory causes (43,1 per cent) followed by low birth weight (19.3 per cent) and infection (12.9 per cent) and Tragante (2009) in a Neonatal Intensive Care Unit at a university hospital in São Paulo with infectious diseases (32 per cent), followed by congenital surgical pathologies (19 per cent).

It was noted that 106 (60.22%) neonates admitted to the labour ward were positive for infection, with a positive culture for bloodstream infection in 51 (48.11%) and the prevalent agent was Klebsiella *sp* in 28 (26.41%) followed by Candida *sp, 22* (20.75%). These findings indicate the poor quality of prenatal care, the importance of continuing education by the CCIH for prevention and hand washing, the overcrowding of NICUs, the failure to provide early enteral nutrition in order to minimise the exuberant neonatal mortality in this study (BITTENCOURT, 2014).

Duarte *et al* (2013) analysed infection in NBs admitted to the NICU in Belo Horizonte/MG, finding a strong association with central catheter infection in very low birth weight premature babies, around 67%. This exposes these patients to a high rate of complications and mortality. Another study that corroborates the association of infection and mortality rates with very low birth weight is the research by Figueiró-Filho *et al* (2014), in addition to relating it to other comorbidities such as pulmonary haemorrhage, hyaline membrane syndrome, pulmonary hypertension, temperature instability, hypoglycaemia and high rates of interventions in the delivery room.

Although neonatal mortality is related to a series of factors of biological origin (antenatal maternal health conditions), social/environmental and care (quality of prenatal care), neonatal death, especially early neonatal death, is the result of immediate neonatal care in the delivery room and neonatal intensive care units. In addition, it is known that if neonates were exposed to the use of antenatal corticosteroids, they would have better birth conditions, with less need for aggressive interventions, better respiratory performance and reduced use of exogenous surfactant, and they would spend less time on mechanical artificial ventilation (BITTENCOURT, 2014).

Given this fact, it can be concluded that some care practices developed in prenatal care, childbirth and the NICU can influence the outcome studied, early neonatal mortality (BITTENCOURT, 2014).

In this sense, it is vitally important to carry out intersectoral interventions aimed at improving women's living conditions and health, both as a right and a need for women themselves, and to guarantee the safe birth and survival of newborns.

In the studies by Calil *et al* (2012) neonatal sepsis is extremely voracious and lethal, and the use of antimicrobials is of fundamental importance in the indicators of discharge, length of stay and hospital resources. Silveira *et al* (2013) reported that sepsis remains one of the main significant causes of early infant morbidity and mortality. Early diagnosis and the judicious use of antibiotic therapy are essential to avoid over-treatment. Blood cultures are the gold standard for identifying the antimicrobial agent to be treated. In the event of a negative culture in a symptomatic neonate, it is advisable to use the shortest course of empirical antibiotic therapy. Treatment should therefore be carefully targeted at the specific microorganism.

Mussi *et al* (2014) reviewed studies outlining the profile of neonatal nosocomial infection, describing the various peculiarities that cause greater susceptibility, survival of the same, as well as the invasive procedures that NBs underwent due to the use of broad-spectrum antimicrobials. Infections affected at least 50 per cent of neonates weighing less than 1500g, causing high mortality. The most common agents were gram-positive bacteria, S. aureus, S. epidermidis, E. coli, K. pneumonia and E. cloacae. Another factor found was resistance to multiple antimicrobial drugs. Mussi created a model epidemiological surveillance programme adapted to the characteristics of the neonatal unit, allowing for the identification of infection outbreaks, the rational use of antibacterials and the application of preventive measures. Unfortunately, this procedure was not observed in the NICUs studied.

As for the figures for discharge and death in the study, the majority had an unfavourable outcome with 142 (80.68%) and only 33 (18.75%) were discharged. There was only one transfer (0.0005%).

Similar data was only found in the study by Granzotto, Fonseca and Lindemann (2012) in a NICU in Pelotas/RS in 2006, where of the 172 newborns admitted, 29 died before reaching one month of life, 20 (68.97%) of which occurred in the first week of life (early neonatal death) and 9 (31.03%) between the first and fourth week of life (late neonatal death).

In the NICUs described in the literature, different results were found, but all of them with higher percentages of discharges and consequently lower percentages of deaths compared to the present study. The studies by Benites and Nunes (2006) in a NICU in Campo Grande/MS in 2002 showed that 77.6% of newborns were discharged, compared to 22.4% who died; Risso and Nascimento (2010) in a NICU in Taubaté/SP between 2005 and 2007 showed that 73.9% of newborns were discharged and 26. 1% died,1 per cent who died, Basso, Neves and Silveira (2012) in a NICU in Rio Grande do Sul with 85.8 per cent discharged and 14.2 per cent who died, Bustamante *et al* (2014) in a NICU in Minas Gerais with 82.4 per cent discharged and 17.6 per cent who died and Lages *et al* (2014) in a NICU in Teresina/PI with 64.1 per cent of neonates discharged and 35.9 per cent who died.

°In a study by Malveira *et al* (2006) on very low birth weight neonates admitted to the FSCMPA Neonatal Unit between 1st January and 30th June 2003, they also found that the main cause of death in these babies was neonatal infection in 78 (39%) of the cases, followed by respiratory distress syndrome (RDS) in 34 (17%) and perinatal anoxia in 7 (3.5%), showing that even after ten years the main cause of death among patients admitted to this institution is still associated with infectious factors. These current findings reflect the urgent need for greater preventive and protective interventions.

Other results have been found in the literature, such as the study by Oliveira, Nunes and Franco (2012) on the morbidity and mortality of NBs in the NICU of a reference hospital for high-risk pregnancies in the interior of Minas Gerais between 2006 and 2010, in which of the 50 NBs who died, 43 (86%) had prematurity as the main cause, followed by respiratory distress syndrome with 29 (58%) and acute respiratory failure with 14%, highlighting the presence of more than one associated morbidity.

Ponciano *et al* (2008) in a NICU in João Pessoa/PB between 2004 and 2008, the main causes of death were infectious diseases in 224 (33.33%), followed by

Cardiopulmonary causes in 162 (24.76%), unidentified causes in 115 (17.14%) and malformations in 67 (10.48%). According to Arrué *et al* (2013), in NICUs in Rio Grande do Sul, prematurity (318 (68%)) was the leading cause of death, followed by cardiopulmonary arrest (219 (47%)) and septicaemia (168 (36%), with most deaths caused by a combination of pathologies.

Furthermore, Basso, Neves and Silveira (2012) found that the main causes of death in NICUs in Rio Grande do Sul were cardiopulmonary arrest, with 135 (27%), followed by prematurity, with 110 (22.2%) and septicaemia with 75 (15.1%). Piesak *et al* (2013) also in NICUs in Rio Grande do Sul between 2002 and 2006 found prematurity with 387 (57.14%) of the cases, septicaemia with 285 (42.41%) and cardiac arrest with 244 (36.16%) as the main causes.

On this subject, Arrué *et al* (2013) describe that neonatal deaths are the result of a close and complex relationship between socio-demographic factors, pregnancy and labour conditions, as well as the characteristics of the newborns.

Also for Lansky *et al* (2014) in a national study on the profile of neonatal mortality and evaluation of care for pregnant women and newborns between 2011 and 2012, they mention that among the causes of neonatal death in the northern region of Brazil, infection 46 (26.9%), congenital malformations 42 (24.5%), prematurity 39 (22. 2%) and asphyxia/hypoxia 23 (13.5%) are among the main causes,2%) and asphyxia/hypoxia 23 (13.5%) are among the main ones, highlighting the great heterogeneity of causes between Brazilian regions and the high mortality rates in the North and Northeast compared to other regions, expressing the need for greater local investment in the organisation and qualification of pre- and perinatal care.

Various authors have stated that mortality in the first six days of life expresses the complex combination of biological, socio-economic and healthcare factors, such as the precariousness of care and the supply of public services for maternal and newborn health. In addition, they emphasise that maternal characteristics such as low schooling, fewer than six prenatal consultations, multiple pregnancies, vaginal delivery, low birth weight and prematurity may be associated with early neonatal mortality (ASSIS, 2008; SOARES; MENEZES, 2010; TRONCO *et al, 2010*).

Corroborating these findings, Gaíva, Bittencourt and Fujimori (2013), regarding the profile of the mothers of newborns who died in the early and late neonatal period, carried out in Cuiabá/MT in 2010, found no differences between them, highlighting, however, that fewer than seven prenatal consultations were carried out, prematurity, low birth weight and an *Apgar score of less* than seven in the first minute of life are characteristics that prevail among early neonatal deaths, indicating the need for greater investment and improvements in the quality of prenatal care at a local level.

According to data from the SUS Informatics Department, neonatal mortality in Brazil from all causes in 2012 was 25.638 deaths, representing the main component of infant mortality, constituting in most cases preventable or treatable deaths, and although it has decreased over the years throughout the country, it is still considered high compared to developed countries, reflecting the quality of prenatal health care, childbirth and the newborn (GOMES, 2004; LAWN et al, 2005; BRASIL, 2009; BRASIL, 2012; DATASUS, 2012).

When correlating the variables low weight, length of stay of less than seven days and use of surfactant in the delivery room with the outcome of discharge/death, there was a strong relationship and an increased risk of death.

The results related to birth weight as a risk factor for neonatal mortality are in line with various studies, where very low birth weight has been found to be strongly associated with unsatisfactory outcomes and death (ARAÚJO *et al,* 2005; GEIB *et al,* 2010; HELENA, SOUSA E SILVA, 2005; OLIVEIRA; GAMA; SILVA, 2010). In the univariate analysis, the study detected a gradually stronger association between low birth weight and the risk of death as birth weight decreased, and this association model was also present in the multivariate analysis and in the final model. A study carried out in Maracanaú, Ceará, to analyse risk factors for infant death, found a statistically significant relationship between live births and low birth weight (OR: 3.16; 95% CI: 1.58;6.35) (SILVA *et al,* 2006).

Barros *et al.* (2006) and Passebon (2006) described the strong association between low birth weight and infant and neonatal death, highlighting the interaction between biological and social factors, recognised in the literature, and reinforcing its maintenance as an isolated criterion for identifying children vulnerable to death.

A prospective cohort study carried out by Castro and Leite (2007), which included all live newborns with a birth weight of 1,500g or less in all maternity hospitals with a neonatal ICU in Fortaleza, reported that the deaths of very low birth weight newborns accounted for approximately 189/42% of total infant mortality. Improving care for these patients in order to reduce infant mortality is one of the fundamental characteristics of the current epidemiological scenario in the municipality.

In contrast to the results of this study, Soares *et al* (2010) reported a mortality rate of low birth weight NBs, with averages of 21% to 34% of discharges due to death in public hospitals in Rio de Janeiro, much lower than that found.

Gonçalves *et al* (2015) traced the trend of neonatal deaths in Salvador from 1996 to 2012, and found that in the Bahian capital, caesarean section, lack of antenatal care and low weight progressively increased the chances of death in neonatal units.

Logistic regression showed that low birth weight, a length of stay of less than seven days and the administration of surfactant in the delivery room increased the chances of death.

Prigenzi (2008) found similar results to the present study. However, the study by Duarte and Mendonça (2005) disagreed, presenting male gender, maternal haemorrhage, the use of mechanical ventilation and birth weight as risk factors for neonatal death in very low birth weight NBs. However, it should be considered that the factors associated with newborn mortality vary according to the characteristics of the population studied, care practices, methodology and study period.

In 2002, the World Health Organisation estimated that 30% to 40% of neonatal deaths were associated with infection, concluding that it was responsible for 1.4 to 1.9 million deaths/year or 3900 to 5200 deaths/day worldwide. The results of this study confirm that the outlook for infections remains bleak for very low birth weight premature babies.

It should be borne in mind that the smaller the premature baby, the more complex the care required for their survival and the more costly their treatment in the ICU will be

and relatively restricted access due to the scarcity of beds, especially in public hospitals. This raises concerns about the cost-effectiveness of the neonatal ICU, especially at the limits of viability. There should be a critical assessment of the results obtained in each service, with a view to knowing its limits and optimising the use of the technological resources available today, in order to guarantee the quality and availability of neonatal care (Prigenzi 2008).

It can be seen that the interaction of the professionals who work in the multidisciplinary team in ICUs can never be seen as routine, continuing education, humanisation and commitment must be individualised, because the neonate, especially the premature infant, has no voice and needs constant care, so that the outcome is discharge home.

CHAPTER 8

PRODUCT

Procedure steps

1- Standardisation

This SOP - Implementation of a multiprofessional bedside visit complies with RDC Resolution No. 7 of 24 February 2010. Session III, Art. 4° , XXII. Routine: comprises the description of the steps taken to carry out an activity or operation, usually involving more than one agent. It encourages planning and rationalisation of the activity, avoids improvisation, as it defines in advance the agents who will be involved, allowing them to train their actions, thus eliminating or minimising errors. They allow for continuity in the actions carried out, as well as providing support for evaluating each one in particular. Routines are unique to each location.

2-Objectives

The aim of the routine multiprofessional visit is to improve and facilitate communication between the professionals in the NICU's multidisciplinary team, exchanging information and optimising treatment. It also aims to draw up joint guidelines in order to help reduce the morbidity and mortality of newborns admitted to the NICUs of the Santa Casa de Misericórdia do Pará Foundation (FSCMPA).

Obeying the precepts of systematised care, which are: Data collection, diagnosis, planning, implementation of multi-professional care and evaluation of the results obtained.

3-Description of the multi-professional visit routine

The routine multi-professional visit will take place every Tuesday and Thursday, in the late morning (11am-12pm), at the bedside, with the participation of the following NICU professionals: the doctor (diarist), the doctor (on call), the doctor (HICU), the two nurses, the physiotherapist, the five nursing technicians, the speech therapist, the occupational therapist, the nutritionist, the psychologist, the pharmacist and the social worker.

The newborns' information will be presented and discussed with the aim of drawing up guidelines to be carried out as soon as possible. The following information will be provided: History of mother and NB, use and days of medication, neuropsychomotor status, haemodynamics (vital signs), respiratory pattern, skin condition, infectious aspects, laboratory and radiological results for the week, nutritional aspects, psychosocial aspects/family humanisation and preventive and palliative measures if necessary.This information will be written down on a check-list sheet of its own, which will contain all the items already mentioned, and next to them the targets that must be achieved. If they are not achieved, they must be justified in writing. In the event of delays in the scheduled procedures, an *Event Notification* will be created and forwarded along with copies of the checklist to the FSCMPA management and board for possible resolution.

4- Benefits of routine

With the routine in place, decisions will be made more confidently regarding the wellbeing of each baby, thus enabling the formulation of personalised and effective conduct.

Optimising working time and improving the quality of care, with the hope of reducing the length of stay in the NICU, hospital costs and reducing morbidity and mortality.

1.1 - CHECK LIST - MULTIPROFESSIONAL VISIT

Patient:				Date of Birth:		
Registration:		NICU:		Date of hospitalisation:		
Weight:		Sex:		Bed:		
Diagnosis:						
Bundles		Date:			Targets:	Obs:
		Yes	No	NA		
CVC	Use of a central venous catheter? Date of insertion:					
	Use of a peripheral venous catheter? Date of insertion:					
	Was an X-ray performed to check the position of the catheter?					
	Signs of hyperaemia or infiltration?					
	Signs of obstruction?					
	Was the dressing changed with sterile transparent semi-permeable film after 7 days?					
SVD	Use of a delayed bladder catheter? Date of insertion:					
	Is the drainage system closed?					
	Is the volume of urine below 2/3 of the level of the collection bag?					
	Signs of obstruction?					
	Physiological appearance of urine?					
PAV	On mechanical ventilation? Start date:					
	PaO2/FiO2 < 300?					
	Can you start weaning from mechanical ventilation?					
	Date: Success weaning from MV					
	Chest X-ray? Change:					
	Suitable cradle position? (raised 45°)					
	TOT number: TOT setting:					
	Signs of obstruction?					
	Physiological appearance of tracheal secretion?					
	Changing the circuit every 7 days?					
	Use of sedation? Type:					

Sedation	Sedation on target?					
	Interruption of sedation?					
	Active and reactive in bed?					
DVA	Use of vasoactive drugs? Type:					
	DVA within target?					
	PAM within the normal range?					
	DVA interruption?					
TEV	Prophylaxis for venous thromboembolism?					
Nutrition	Gastric prophylaxis?					
	Use of an orogastric tube?					
	Can it be nourished?					
	For drainage? Appearance of secretion:					
	Need a replacement?					
	Full Expected Volume?					
	Performing oral hygiene?					
	As a precaution? Like:					
	Which micro-organism?					
ATB	Use of antibiotics?					
	Which antibiotic?					
	Can antibiotics be removed?					
	Antibiotic dose adjustment necessary?					
Cort	Use of corticosteroids?					
	Can corticosteroids be stopped?					
BH	What is the water balance?					
GLI	Adequate glycaemic control?					
Fabric	Skin appearance?					
	Skin discontinuity?					
	Type of dressing					
	Appropriate use of fasteners? Type:					
	Any drains? Like:					
CCIH	Culture in demand? Date:					
Physio	Do you do respiratory physiotherapy?					
	Do you do motor physiotherapy?					
	Any restrictions? Like:					
Family	Did you welcome them?					
	Breastfeeding?					
	Carrying out the kangaroo method?					

1.2 - EVENT NOTIFICATION FORM

Event Notification

Identification of the Notifier	
Name:	
Role:	NICU:
Contact	

Type of Notification		Prescription		Intercurrence with the patient		Diet
		Medicament		Equipment/product/material		Tests
		Medical visit		Surgical Procedures		Transport and transfer
		Employee event		Others		

Date of registration:	Event Date:
NICU where the event took place:	
Event Description	

CHAPTER 9

CONCLUSION

According to the methodology used and the results obtained in this study on the avoidability of neonatal death in very low birth weight premature infants admitted to the intensive care units of a teaching hospital in the North, it can be concluded that:

1- The average length of stay was 13 days. The vast majority of babies were hospitalised for no more than seven days.
2- There was a relationship between weight, length of stay and use of medication with the mortality rate and the outcome of discharge, revealing a strong relationship between lower weight and shorter length of stay in ICUs with the outcome of death.
3- The lower the weight, the more resources were used, not increasing the length of stay in the units and/or decreasing the mortality rate of the newborns.
4- Most of the low-birth-weight patients hospitalised used some form of ventilatory support, the most common being mechanical ventilation using an oro-tracheal tube. However, this did not increase the length of stay of the neonates
5- Bloodstream infection was prevalent among the newborns, with Klebsiella *sp* being the main agent. The most commonly used antimicrobials were the 1st generation, showing no correlation with the mortality rate.
6- It was therefore proposed that a multi-professional routine be implemented, with the aim of improving results in the units and encouraging all professionals to take part in behaviour.

Given these findings, we can see the fragility of health services in relation to the care of low birth weight newborns in intensive care units. In addition, it is necessary to update routines, continue education and studies to improve care according to the particularities of this population. This will enable newborns to survive with better outcomes.

BIBLIOGRAPHICAL REFERENCES

ALMAD R, et al. **Changes in cerebral venous prostanoids during midazolam- induced cerebrovascular hypotension in newborn piglets.** Crit Care Med28:2429, 2008

ALVES, C. S. P.; OLIVEIRA, M. L.; SANTOS, M. L.; MEREY, L. S. F.; ALENCAR, S. P.; CARREGARO, R. L.; TOLEDO, A. M. **The influence of prematurity on respiratory complications in neonates.** Braz. J. Phys. Ther., v.16, n. 9, Supl. 2, p.265-265, 2012.

ARAÚJO, B. F. et al. **Mortality study of newborns admitted to the neonatal ICU of the**

General Hospital of Caxias do Sul, Rio Grande do Sul. Rev. Bras. Saúde Matem. Infant. Recife, v. 5, n. 4, p. 463-9, Oct./Dec. 2005.

ARRUÉ, A. M.; NEVES, E. T.; SILVEIRA, A.; PIESZAK, G. M. **Characterisation of the morbidity and mortality of newborns admitted to the Neonatal Intensive Care Unit.** Rev. Enferm., Santa Maria, v. 3, n. 1, p. 86-92, jan./abr., 2013.

ASSIS, H. M. **Early neonatal morbidity and mortality profiles:** a study for the Odete Valadares Maternity Hospital in Belo Horizonte (MG), 2001-2006. 2008. Dissertation (Master's in Demography) - Federal University of Minas Gerais, Belo Horizonte, 2008.

AZEVEDO, G. D.; FREITAS JÚNIOR, R. A. O.; FREITAS, A. K. M. S. O.; ARAÚJO, A. C. P. F.; SOARES, E. M. M.; MARANHÃO, T. M. O. **Effect of Maternal Age on Perinatal Outcomes. Original Articles.** Rev. Bras. Gynaecol. Obstet., v. 24, n. 3, 2002.

BARBOSA, A. P.; CUNHA, A. J. L. A.; CARVALHO, E. R. M.; PORTELLA, A. F.; ANDRADE, M. P. F.; BARBOSA, M. C. M. **Neonatal and paediatric intensive care in Rio de Janeiro: bed distribution and equity analysis.** Rev. Assoe. Med. Bras., n. 48, v. 4, p. 303-311, 2002.

BARBOSA, A. P. **Neonatal and paediatric intensive care in Brazil: the ideal, the real and the possible.** J. Pediatr., Rio de Janeiro, v. 80, n. 6, p. 437- 438, nov./dez. 2004.
BARBOSA, A. L.; CHAVES, E. M. C.; CAMPOS, A. C. S. **Characterisation of newborns on mechanical ventilation in a Neonatal Unit.** Rev. Rene, Fortaleza, v. 8, n. 2, p. 35-40, May/Aug.2007.

BARROS, F. C. et al. **Maternal and child health in Pelotas. Rio Grande do Sul, Brazil: main conclusions from the comparison of the studies of the 1982 to 1993 cohorts.** Cad. Saude Publica, v. 12, n. 1, p. 87-92, 2006.

BASSO, C. G.; NEVES, E. T.; SILVEIRA, A. **Association between prenatal care and neonatal morbidity.** Redalyc, Santa Catarina, v. 21, n. 2, p. 269-276, April-June 2012.

BERGMAN I, et al. **Reversible neurologic abnormalities associated with prolonged intravenous midazolam and fentanyl administration.** J Paediatr 119:644,2009

BITTENCOURT, R. M.; GAIVA, M. A. M. **Early neonatal mortality related to clinical interventions.** Rev. Bras. Enferm., v. 67, n.2, p. 195-201, 2014.

BONITA, R.; BEAGLEHOLE, R.; KJELLSTRÔM, T. **Epidemiologia básica/** Basic epidem**iology**. 2ª ed. - São Paulo: Santos, 2010. 213p.

BRAZIL. **Prenatal care.** Ministry of Health. Health Care Secretariat. Department of Programmatic and Strategic Actions, Brasília, DF, 2000.

. **Newborn health care:** guide for health professionals, v. 1. General Care. Brasília, DF, 2011. (Series A. Standards and Technical Manuals). A

. **Newborn health care: a** guide for health professionals, v. 3. Respiratory, cardiocirculatory, metabolic, neurological, orthopaedic and dermatological problems. Brasília, DF, 2011. (Series A. Standards and Technical Manuals). B

. **High-risk pregnancy:** technical manual. 5. ed. Brasília, DF, 2010. A

. **Neonatal IMCI manual** / Ministry of Health, Pan American Health Organisation. - 3ª . ed. Brasília, DF, 2012, 228 p. Available at: <www.saude.gov.br>. Accessed on: 09 Sep. 2013. **BRAZIL 2012 A**

. **Manual de vigilância do óbito infantil e fetal e do Comité de Prevenção do Óbito Infantil e Fetal.** 2. ed. Secretaria de Vigilância em Saúde. Health Care Secretariat. Brasília, DF, 2009, 96p. A

. **Information note 2010.** Expansion and qualification of neonatal ICU beds in the northeast and legal Amazon. Brasília, DF, 14 September 2010. Available at: http://portal.saude.gov.br. Accessed on: 23 January 2014. B

^**Portaria n° 3.432,** of 12 August 1998. Available at http://portal.anvisa.gov.br. Accessed on: 11 January 2014.

. **Ordinance No. 570,** of I° June 2000. Ministry of Health, Brasília, DF. 2000. Available at: http://bvsms.saude.gov.br. Accessed on: 21 July 2014.

. **Ordinance no. 930,** of 10 May 2012. Ministry of Health, Brasília, DF. 2012. Available at: http://bvsms.saude.gov.br. Accessed on: 11 August 2013.

. **Database medical records:** systematised information for Brazil's health accounts. Ana Cecilia de Sá Campello Faveret (Org.) Brasília: Ipea, 2009. B

. **Proportion of live births with 7 or more prenatal consultations, by year, according to region and mother's schooling.** Rio de Janeiro. Social Determinants of Health

Portal. Observatory on Health Inequities. CEPI- DSS/ENSP/FIOCRUZ; 30 Jan. 2012. B

. **Resolution-RDC no. 7,** of 24 February 2010. Ministry of Health. National Health Surveillance Agency. Provides for the minimum requirements for the operation of Intensive Care Units and other measures. Available at: http://brasilsus.com.br/legislacoes/rdc/102985-7.html. Accessed on: 11 August 2013.

. **Saúde Brasil 2011:** an analysis of the health situation and women's health surveillance. Health Surveillance Secretariat. Department of Health Situation Analysis. Brasília: DF, 2012. 444 p. C

BROWN, M. K.; DIBLASI, R. M. **Mechanical Ventilation of the Premature Neonate.** Respiratory Care, v. 56, n. 9, p. 203-215, sep. 2011.

BURTIN P, et. **Hypotension with midazolam and fentatnyl in the newborn.** Lancet 337:1545, 2007

CASTRO, E. C. M.; LEITE, A. J. M. **Hospital mortality of newborns with birth weight less than or equal to 1,500 g in the municipality of Fortaleza. J.** Pediatr. (Rio J.), Porto Alegre, v. 83, n. 1, p. 27-32, feb. 2007.

CARDOSO, P. O.; ALBERTI, L. R.; PETROIANU, A. Neonatal and maternal morbidity related to the type of delivery. **Ciênc. saúde coletiva,** v.15, n.2, p. 427-435, 2010.

CARMO, C. M. A.; OLIVEIRA, E. M.; PONTES, K. A. E.; MARTINS, T. B.; CABRAL, T. C. G. **Nursing procedures** in the **neonatal ICU** in MOREIRA, M. E. L.; LOPES, J. M. A.; CARALHO, M. (eds). The high-risk newborn: theory and practice of care. Coleção criança, mulher e saúde, Rio de Janeiro: Editora FIOCRUZ, 2004. 564 p. Available at:< http://books.scielo.org/id/wcgvd>. Accessed on: 06 August 2013.

CLOHERTY, J. P.; EICHENWALD, E. C.; STARK, A. R. **Manual of neonatology.** Rio de Janeiro: Guanabara Koogan; 2009.

COELHO, M. A. F.; AMARANTE, S. C. **Main causes of hospitalisation in the Neonatal Intensive Care Unit, in July 2010, in a private hospital in the city of Cascavel.** Dissertation (Final course work in Nursing) - Assis Gurgacs College, 2010.

CUNHA, A. A; FERNANDES, D. S; MELO, P. F.; GUEDES, M. H. Factors Associated with Perinatal Asphyxia. **Rev. Bras. Gynaecol. Obstet.,** v. 26, n. 10, 2004.

DEVER, A. G. E.; CHAMPAGNE, F. A **epidemiologia na administração dos serviços de saúde** / Epidemiology in health **services** management. São Paulo: Pioneira, 1988. 394 p.

DRUMMOND, S; SOUZA, T. S.; LIMA, F. G.; VIEIRA, A. A. Correlation between the use of antenatal corticotherapy, resuscitation and mortality of very low birth weight premature newborns. **Rev. Bras. Gynaecol. Obstet.,** v.36, n.5, p. 211-215, 2014.

DUARTE JLB, MENDONÇA GAS. **Factors associated with neonatal death in very low birth weight infants in four maternity hospitals in the city of Rio de Janeiro.** Cad Saúde Pública. 2005; 21: 181-91.

FILHO, N. A.; BARRETO, M. L. **Epidemiologia & saúde: fundamentos, métodos, aplicações.** [Reimpr.] - Rio de Janeiro: Guanabara Koogan, 2012.

FILIZOLA, A. C.; JULIANO, Y.; ARMOND, J. E.; BERTAGNON, J. R. Newborns in the Neonatal Intensive Care Unit: The importance of resuscitation in the delivery room. **Rev. Bras. Ciênc. da Saúde,** v. 30, n. 22, Oct/Dec 2009.

FREDDI, N. A.; PROENÇA FILHO, J. O.; FIORI, H. H. Therapy with exogenous pulmonary surfactant in paediatrics. **J. Pediatr.** v. 79, supl. 2, p. 205-212, 2003.

UNITED NATIONS CHILDREN'S FUND (UNICEF). **State of the World's Children 2008,** Brazil Notebook. Brazil, DF, January 2008, 64p. Available at: http://www.unicef.org.br. Accessed on: 10 August 2013.

. **State of the World's Children 2009.** Available at: http://www.unicef.org/brazil. Accessed on: 17 August 2013.

GOMES, M. A. M. **Organisation of perinatal care** in **Brazil** in MOREIRA, M. E. L.; LOPES, J. M. A.; CARALHO, M. (eds). The high-risk newborn: theory and practice of care. Coleção criança, mulher e saúde, Rio de Janeiro: FIOCRUZ, 2004. 564 p.

GAÍVA, M. A. M; BITTENCOURT, R. M.; FUJIMORI, E. Early and late neonatal death: profile of mothers and newborns. **Rev. Gaúcha Enferm.,** v. 34, n. 4, p. 91- 97, 2013.

GEIB, L. T. C. et al. **Social and biological determinants of infant mortality in a population-based cohort in Passo Fundo, Rio Grande do Sul.** Ciência & Saúde Coletiva. Rio Grande do Sul. v. 15, n.2, p. 363-70, 2010.

GRANZOTTO, J. A.; FONSECA, S. S.; LINDEMANN, F. L. Factors related to neonatal mortality in a neonatal intensive care unit in southern Brazil. **Revista da AMRIGS,** Porto Alegre, v. 56, v.l, p. 57-62, jan.-mar, 2012.

GRANZOTTO, J. A.; MOTA, D. M.; REAL, R. F.; DIAS, C. M.; TEIXEIRA, R. F.; FILHO, J.C.M.; TIECHER, G. B.; PILECCO, A. J. L.; GONÇALVES, E. R. Analysis of the epidemiological profile of admissions to a neonatal intensive care unit. **Revista da AMRIGS,** Porto Alegre, v. 56, n.4, p. 304-307, Oct-Dec, 2012.
GONÇALVES-FERRI, W.A; MARTINEZ, F. E. Nasal CPAP in the delivery room for newborns with extremely low birth weight in a hospital in a developing country. **Brazilian Journal of Medicine and Biological Research,** v. 17, n. 46, p. 892-896, 2013.

HARTE GJ, et al. **Haemodynamic responses and population pharmacokinetics of midazolam following administration to ventilated, preterm neonates.** J Paediatr Child Health 133:335,2009

JACQZ-AIGRAIN E, et al. **Pharmacokinetics of midazolam during continuous infusion in critically ill neonates.** J Clin Pharmacol 42:329, 2009

JOHNSTON, C.; CARVALHO, W. B.; BARBOSA, A. P.; HORIGOSHI, N. K.; ZANETTI , N. M.; MELO, A.P. L.; BARCELLOS, P. G.; CARR, A. M. G.; SARMENTO, G. J. V.; REBELLO, C. M.; I Consenso Brasileiro de ventilação mecânica em pediatria e neonatologia. Brazilian Intensive Care Medicine Association; Brazilian Paediatric Society, 2008.

JOHNSTON, C.; ZANETTI, N. M.; COMARU, T.; RIBEIRO, S. N. S.; ANDRADE, L. B.; SANTOS, S. L. L. I Recomendação Brasileira de Fisioterapia respiratória em Unidade de Terapia Intensiva Pediátrica e Neonatal. **Rev. Bras. Ter. Intensiva,** v. 24, n.2, p.l 19-129, 2012.

KAMADA L; ROCHA, S. M. M.; BARBEIRA, C.B.S. Hospitalisations in neonatal intensive care units in Brazil - 1998-2001. **Rev. Latino-am Enfermagem,** v. 11, n. 4, p. 436-443, jul.-ago., 2003.

KAMADA I.; ROCHA, S. M. M.; BARBEIRA, C.B.S. Hospitalisations in neonatal intensive care units in Brazil - 1998-2001. **Rev. Latino-am Enfermagem,** v. 11, n. 4, p. 436-443, jul.-ago., 2003.

KIRPALANI, H.; MILLAR, D.; LEMYRE, B.; YODER, B. A; CHIU, A.; Roberts, R. S. A Trial Comparing Noninvasive Ventilation Strategies in Preterm Infants. **N. Engl J Med,** v. 369,

n. 15, p.7, Aug. 2013.
LAMARCA, M. V.G. **Prenatal care in Brazil: a question of supply, access or maternal schooling?** Rio de Janeiro: Social Determinants of Health Portal. Observatory on Health Inequities. CEPI-DSS/ENSP/FIOCRUZ, 28 May 2012. Accessed on: 23 July 2014. Available at: http://dssbr.org/site/2012/05/atencao-pre- natal-no-brasil-uma-questao-de-oferta-de-accesso-ou-de-escolaridade-matema/.

LAWN, J. E.; COUSENS, S.; ZUPAN, J.; Lancet Neonatal Survival Steering Team. 4 million neonatal deaths: when? where? why? **Lancet,** v. 365, n. 9462, p. 891-900, mar. 2005.

LEÃO, E. V.V.; VIEIRA, M. E. B.; PEREIRA, S. A. Profile of CPAP use in the neonatal ICU and the role of the physiotherapist. **Rev. Movimenta,** v. 6, n. 1, p. 386- 397, 2013.

LOPES, J. M. The use of "CPAP" in neonatal ventilatory assistance. **J. Pediatr,** v. 76, n.5, p. 329-330, 2000.

MACHADO, L. C.; PASSINI, R. J.; ROSA, I. R. M. Late prematurity: a systematic review. **J. Pediatr,** Rio de Janeiro, v. 90, n. 3, p. 221-231, 2014.

MALVEIRA, S. S.; MORAES, A. N; CHERMONT, A.G.; COSTA, D. L. F.; SILVA, T. F. Very low birth weight newborns in a reference hospital. **Rev. Para. Med.,** v. 20, n.l, p. 41-46, 2006.

MENEGUEL, J. F. et al. Antenatal treatment with corticosteroids for preterm neonates: impact on the incidence of respiratory distress syndrome and intra-hospital mortality. **J. Med.,** São Paulo, v.121, n. 2, p. 45-52, 2003.

MIYOSHI, M. H.; GUINSBURG, R. **Ventilatory support in newborn respiratory distress syndrome.** In I Brazilian Consensus on mechanical ventilation in paediatrics and neonatology. AMIB-Brazilian intensive care medicine association, 2008. Accessed on: 14 January 2014.

MOREIRA, M. E. L.; LOPES, J. M. A.; CARALHO, M. (eds). **The high-risk newborn:** theory and practice of care. Child, woman and health collection. Rio de Janeiro: FIOCRUZ, 2004. 564 p.
MOREIRA, M. E. L.; LOPES, J. M. A.; CARALHO, M. (eds). **The high-risk newborn:** theory and practice of care. Child, woman and health collection. Rio de Janeiro: FIOCRUZ, 2004. 564 p.

OLIVEIRA, E. F. V.; GAMA, S. G. N.; SILVA, C. M. F. P. **Teenage pregnancy and other**

risk factors for foetal and infant mortality in the municipality of Rio de Janeiro, Brazil. Cad. saúde Publ. v. 26, n.3, p. 567-78, mar. 2010.

PAIM, J. S. Epidemiologia e planejamento: a recomposição das práticas epidemiológicas na gestão do SUS. **Ciênc. saúde coletiva,** v. 8, n. 2, p. 557-567, 2003.

RISSO, S. P.; NASCIMENTO, L. F. C. Risk factors for death in a neonatal intensive care unit, using the survival analysis technique. **Rev. bras. ter. intensiva,** v.22, n.l, p. 19-26, 2010.

ROBERTS, C. L; BADGERY-PARKER, T.; ALGERT, C. S; BOWEN, J. R; NASSAR, N. Trends in use of neonatal CP AP: a population-based study. **Pediatrics,** v. 11, n. 89, p.1-7, 2011.

ROCHA. R; OLIVEIRA C.; SILVA, D. K. F.; BONFIM, C. Neonatal mortality and avoidability: an analysis of the epidemiological profile. **Rev. enferm.,** Rio de Janeiro, v. 19, n. l,p. 114-20, jan-mar 2011.

ROSA, M. K. O.; GAÍVA. M. A. M. Qualidade na atenção hospitalar ao recém-nascido. **Rev. Rene,** Fortaleza, v. 10, n. 1, p. 1-165, jan.-mar. 2009.

SALUSTIANO, E. M. A; CAMPOS, J. A. D. B; IBIDI, S. M; RUANO, R.; ZUGAIB, M. Low Apgar scores at 5 minutes in a low risk population: maternal and obstetrical factors and postnatal outcome. **Rev. Assoe. Med. Bras.,** v. 58, n. 5, p. 587-593, 2012.

SANTOS, G. H. N.; MARTINS, M. G.; SOUSA, M. S.; BATALHA, S. J. C. Impact of maternal age on perinatal outcomes and mode of delivery. **Rev. Bras. Ginecol. Obstet.,** v.31, n.7, p. 326-334, 2009.

SANTOS, L. M.; PASQUINI, V. Z. The importance of the *Apgar score.* **Rev. Enferm,** UNISA, v. 10, n. 1, p. 39-43. 2009.

SCOCHI, C. G. S.; COSTA, I. A R.; YAMANAKA, N. M. A. Historical evolution of newborn care: an overview. **Acta Paul. Enf.,** São Paulo, v. 9, p. 91-101,1996. Special issue.

SILVA, C. F. et al. **Risk factors for infant mortality in a municipality in the Northeast of Brazil: linkage between databases of live births and infant deaths - 2000 to 2002.** Rev. bras. epidemiol., São Paulo, v. 9, n. 1, p. 69-80, mar. 2006.

SILVA, C. F.; LEITE, A. J. M.; ALMEIDA, N. M. G. S.; LEON, A. C. M. P.;

OLOFIN, I. **Factors associated with neonatal death in high-risk newborns: a multicentre study in High-Risk Neonatal Units in the Brazilian Northeast.** Cad. Saúde Pública, Rio de Janeiro, v. 30, n. 2, p. 355-368, feb. 2014.

SILVA, Z. P. et al. **Characteristics of live births, mothers and early neonatal mortality in the Metropolitan Region of São Paulo, Brazil.** Cad. Saúde Pública, Rio de Janeiro, v. 25, n. 9, p. 1981-89, Sep. 2009.

BRAZILIAN SOCIETY OF PAEDIATRICS. **Ratio of the number of neonatal ICU beds per 1000 live births.** Estimate of the need for neonatal ICU beds in Brazil, 08/05/2012. Available at: http://www.sbp.com.br. Accessed on: 26 August 2013.

. **Neonatal resuscitation in the delivery room:** Scientific document of the Neonatal Resuscitation Programme of the Brazilian Society of Paediatrics, 2012. Available at: http://www.sbp.com.br. Accessed on: 26 August 2014.

SOARES, E. S; MENEZES, G. M. S. Factors associated with early neonatal mortality: analysing the situation at the local level. **Epidemiol. Serv. Saúde,** v.19, n.l, p. 51-60, 2010.

TADIELO, B. Z.; NEVES, E. T.; ARRUÉ A. M.; SILVEIRA, A.; RIBEIRO, A. C.; TRONCO, C. S.; NEVES, A. T.; WEIS, P. S. C. Morbidity and mortality of newborns in neonatal intensive care in southern Brazil. **Rev. Soc. Bras. Nurs.** São Paulo, v.13, n.l, p. 7-12, jul. 2013.

TEIXEIRA, M.A.D.; ALCANTARA, E.C. Analysis of the use of surfactant, ventilatory support, length of hospital stay and number of deaths in newborns from different gestational ages. **Rev. Bras. Fisioter.,** v. 14, Supl 1, p. 478-486, 2010.

THOMPSON, M. H.; KHOT, A. S. Impact of neonatal intensive care. **Archives of Disease in Childhood,** v. 60, p. 213-214,1985.

TRONCO, C. S.; PAULA, C. C.; PADOIN, S. M. M.; LANGENDORF, T. F. Analysis of scientific production on care for low birth weight newborns in ICUs. Rev. **Gaúcha Enferm.** Porto Alegre, v. 31, n. 3, p. 575-83, sep. 2010.

VAN STRAATEN HL, et al. **Comparison of the effect of midazolam or vecuronium on blood pressure and cerebral blood flow velocity in the premature newborn.** Dev Pharmacol Ther 19:191, 2008

WAISMAN D, et al. **Myoclonic movements in very low birth weight premature infants associated with midazolam intravenous bolus administration.** Paediatrics 104:3,2008

XIMENES, F. M. A.; OLIVEIRA, M. C. R. The influence of maternal age on perinatal conditions. **Rev. Bras. Gynaecol. Obstet.,** v.17, n. 2, p. 56-60, 2004.

ANNEXES

ANNEX A (OPINION OF THE TEACHING AND RESEARCH COMMITTEE)

FUNDAÇÃO SANTA CASA DE MISERICÓRDIA DO PARÁ - FSCMPA

PARECER CONSUBSTANCIADO DO CEP

DADOS DO PROJETO DE PESQUISA

Título da Pesquisa: Caracterização dos recém-nascidos de baixo peso internados nas Unidades de Terapia Intensiva de um Hospital Escola na Região Norte

Pesquisador: Fabiano Jose da Silva Boulhosa

Área Temática:

Versão: 1

CAAE: 44804615.4.0000.5171

Instituição Proponente: Fundação Santa Casa de Misericórdia do Para

Patrocinador Principal: Financiamento Próprio

DADOS DO PARECER

Número do Parecer: 1.074.331

Data da Relatoria: 22/05/2015

Apresentação do Projeto:

Os Recém-nascidos prematuros e de baixo peso representam, entre a população neonatal, os grupos mais vulneráveis ao óbito, alem de gerar um tempo de internação maior nas unidades hospitalares. O baixo peso ao nascer e os fatores que estão associados a essa condição são fundamentais no planejamento de programas e politicas publicas de saúde e nutrição. O estudo visa conheça o perfil destes usuários internados nas Unidades de Terapia Intensiva visando dispor de dados que permitam o melhor planejamento ao atendimento global do paciente. Esse conhecimento faz-se necessário, uma vez que a partir do mesmo pode-se traçar estratégias de melhor assistir os indivíduos nela internados, avaliando, o prognósticos, os efeitos da terapêutica implementada, bem como fatores de riscos que os vulnerabilizam. Trata-se de um projeto de pesquisa analitico, comparativo e retrospectivo, do perfil de recém-nascidos prematuros menores ou igual a 1.500g internados nas Unidades de Terapia Intensiva de um único centro hospitalar no município de Belém – Pará, no período de janeiro a dezembro de 2014.

Objetivo da Pesquisa:

Analisar o perfil clínico, epidemiológico e sócio-demográfico de recém-nascidos prematuros menor ou igual a 1.500 g internados nas Unidades de Terapia Intensiva (UTI's) de janeiro a dezembro de 2014

Endereço: Rua Oliveira Belo, 395
Bairro: umarizal **CEP:** 66.050-380
UF: PA **Município:** BELEM
Telefone: (91)4009-2264 **Fax:** (91)4009-0326 **E-mail:** comite.eticafscmpa@yahoo.com.br

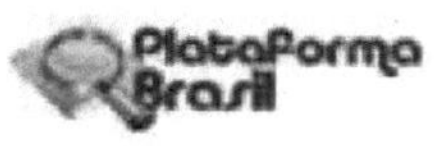

Avaliação dos Riscos e Benefícios:

Os riscos serão mínimos pois não haverá intervenção dos pesquisadores e a coleta de dados será no departamento de arquivo do hospital

Benefícios: Através do estudo será possível conhecer as possíveis falhas no tratamento e posteriormente, traçar o desenvolvimento de estratégias mais específicas e eficazes no manejo do recém-nascido, através de protocolo de visita multiprofissional beira-leito nas UTI's.

Comentários e Considerações sobre a Pesquisa:

Estudo com mérito científico com desenho metodológico adequado e atendendo aos aspectos éticos necessários ao desenvolvimento da pesquisa

Considerações sobre os Termos de apresentação obrigatória:

Todos os termos necessários foram apresentados de forma adequada

Recomendações:

Não há recomendações

Conclusões ou Pendências e Lista de Inadequações:

Trabalho atende aos critérios de aprovação

Situação do Parecer:

Aprovado

Necessita Apreciação da CONEP:

Não

Considerações Finais a critério do CEP:

Aprovado de acordo com parecer do relator.

BELEM, 22 de Maio de 2015

Assinado por:
Solange Carneiro Antonelli
(Coordenador)

Endereço: Rua Oliveira Belo, 395
Bairro: umarizal CEP: 66.050-380
UF: PA Município: BELEM
Telefone: (91)4009-2264 Fax: (91)4009-0328 E-mail: comite.eticafscmpa@yahoo.com.br

ANNEX B (DATA USE CONSENT FORM)

CONSENT FORM FOR THE USE OF DATA FROM ARCHIVES AND MEDICAL RECORDS
Project title: Characterisation of low birth weight newborns admitted to the Intensive Care Units of a Teaching Hospital in the Northern Region. **Researcher responsible:** Fabiano José da Silva Boulhosa **Participating researchers:** Fabiano José da Silva Boulhosa Aurimery Gomes Chermont **Database:** Medical and Statistical Service of the Santa Casa de Misericórdia Foundation of Pará (SAME/FSCMPA). **The researchers in the project identified above undertake to:** I. Preserving the privacy of the patients whose data will be collected; II. Ensure that the information will be used solely and exclusively for the execution of the project in question; III. Ensure that the information will only be disclosed anonymously, and that no initials or any other indications that could identify the research subject will be used. Belém, from
Fabiano José da Silva Boulhosa
Aurimery Gomes Chermont

ANNEX C (DATA COLLECTION FORM)

Ficha: Nome: Registro:
Dados de Admissão
Idade da Mãe: (10 a 19 – 01; 20 a 34- 02; ≥35 – 03)
Data da Internação:
Data de Nascimento:
Procedência:
Sexo: (Masculino – 01; Feminino – 02)
Idade Gestacional: (>28 sem – 01; 28 a 31 – 02; 32 a 36 – 03; 37 a 41- 04; < 42 sem – 05)
Peso:
Consulta pré-natal: (Sim – 01; Não- 02)
Numero de Consultas: (1 a 5 consultas – 01; < 6 – 02)
Tipo de Parto: (Vaginal – 01; Cesariano- 02)
Intercorrencias pré-natal:
(Sim – 01; Não- 02)
Surfactante: (Sim - 01; Não-02)
DVA: (Sim- 01; Não-02)
Qual DVA:
Tempo de DVA:
Sedação: (Sim- 01; Não-02)
Tempo de Sedação:
Corticoide antenatal: (Sim-01; Não-02)
Recurso Ventilátorio: (Sim-01; Não- 02)
Qual recurso Ventilatorio: (IOT-01; VNI-02; HOOD-03; O2 – 04)
Drenos: (Sim-01; Não-02)
Local do Dreno:

Dados de Alta
UTI:
Dias de UTI: (≤ 7-01; 8 a 14 – 02; 15 a 21- 03; 22 a 28 -04; ≥ 28 -05)
Complicações durante a internação: (Sim – 01; Não- 02)
Complicação Respiratória:
Complicação Hemodinâmica:
Abordagem cirúrgica: (Sim – 01; Não -02)
Qual Cirurgia:
Hemodiálise: (Sim – 01; Não – 02)
Dias de hemodiálise:
Infecção durante a internação: (Sim – 01; Não – 02)
Local infectado:
Culturas: (Traqueal – 01; Hemocultura – 02; Urocultura – 03; Swab – 04; LCR- 05; Outro- 06)
Agente(s):
Antibiótico: (Sim – 01; Não – 02)
Qual antibiótico:
Tempo de uso do antibiótico:
Tempo de Ventilação Mecânica:
Tempo de VNI:
Tempo de Drenos:
TQT: (Sim – 01; Não –02)
Tipo de alta: (Enfermaria – 01; Transferência extra-hospitalar – 02; Óbito – 03)
Cause de Óbito:
Retorno à UTI em 48h: (Sim – 01 ; Não -02)
Falha da Alta:

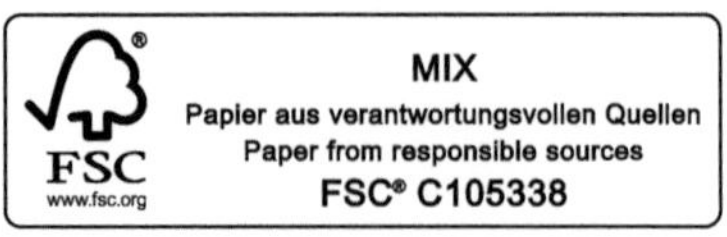

Printed by Books on Demand GmbH, Norderstedt / Germany